DEATH TOUCH

TOUCH

THE SCIENCE BEHIND THE LEGEND OF DIM-MAK

Michael Kelly, D.O.
Foreword by Erle Montaigue

Paladin Press · Boulder, Colorado

This book is dedicated to my son, David.

Death Touch: The Science Behind the Legend of Dim-Mak
by Michael Kelly, D.O.

Copyright © 2001 by Michael Kelly, D.O.

ISBN 1-58160-281-2
Printed in the United States of America

Published by Paladin Press, a division of
Paladin Enterprises, Inc.
Gunbarrel Tech Center
7077 Winchester Circle
Boulder, Colorado 80301 USA
+1.303.443.7250

Direct inquiries and/or orders to the above address.

Visit our Web site at www.paladin-press.com

Table of
Contents

Disclaimer

T his book is intended to be used as an educational tool to warn the public about the dangers of attacking the dim-mak points. The author and publisher do not take any responsibility for any injuries, harm, or deaths that are the result of someone's using the information contained in this book for other than educational purposes. No one should ever strike, grab, or otherwise attack the dim-mak points or nerves mentioned in this book because doing so can result in great bodily harm or death.

The methods of healing described in this book are presented *for academic study only.* This in no way implies that the author and publisher endorse these methods. The author and publisher take no responsibility for any injuries, harm, or deaths that are the result of someone's attempting to use the healing methods presented in this book for other than educational purposes. Any injuries or illness, whether related to dim-mak or not, should be treated by a licensed physician. Additionally, one should consult a physician before engaging in any physical activity associated with any form of martial arts training.

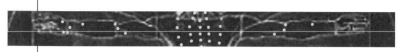

Foreword

I have been associated with Michael Kelly for some time, having published several of his excellent articles in the World Taiji Boxing Association (WTBA) magazine, *Combat & Healing*. Over the years I have known him, I have often thought that he should compile all of his research into a book, which he has now done.

Having read the first finished draft of his manuscript, I am very happy with the outcome. This is not just a bunch of articles but a thoroughly researched and thought out scientific work. For those who are skeptical about dim-mak and need further scientific evidence for the various points and why they work, this book is a must. For those who already know about dim-mak, it is also an essential work because it presents, from a medical point of view, the background of the art and the reasons the points, both singularly and in combination, have their respective effects on the anatomy.

This book is an excellent companion to my two-volume *Encyclopedia of Dim-Mak*.

I can thoroughly recommend this book to all

martial artists. It will enhance their knowledge and also give them ammunition to use in debating with those who perhaps are nonbelievers.

—Erle Montaigue
Master Degree, China
June 13, 2000

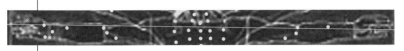

Acknowledgments

I would like to take this opportunity to thank a number of people who helped me with this book. Erle Montaigue not only wrote the foreword but also generously offered his advice and encouragement. I believe that he embodies the true spirit of the martial arts. Karen Petersen is an outstanding editor as well as an exceptional person. Dr. Robert Ehlers graciously allowed me to draw the points on his body and then take photographs of him. I would like to thank Dr. Julie Renda for all of her contributions to this book and for helping me to become a better writer. Finally, I would like to thank my family for their unconditional love and support in all of my endeavors.

Introduction

The martial arts are enjoyed by thousands of people around the world. Many people practice one of the various forms of martial arts for physical fitness or stress reduction. Some learn the arts for more personal reasons such as character development, self-discipline, and confidence. Finally, there are those who study the martial arts for self-defense. The latter is the reason the martial arts were created. In fact, the original intended purpose of the martial arts was to enable one to survive a fight to the death. Through the years, as the need to defend one's life diminished, the focus of training shifted from combat to character development. This was not necessarily a negative change, because many practitioners have derived great benefits from this aspect of the martial arts. However, they are called martial arts because there is a side that deals with fighting. There are some students who are interested in this combat side and wish to study an art that can give them both the development of character and an effective method of combat. Thanks to the efforts of some

1

innovative masters, this combat side is reappearing through the open teaching of dim-mak.

The term *dim-mak* translates into death touch and involves striking acupuncture points to cause injury or death. A component of many different martial arts, dim-mak is also known as kyusho jitsu, vital point attacking, and pressure-point fighting.

Dim-mak is believed to have originated in ancient China and derived from ancient acupuncture theories. According to legend, Zhang Sanfeng who was both a martial artist and acupuncturist, attempted to devise a martial art that focused on attacking the points that were deemed too dangerous for acupuncture. It is believed that he experimented on prisoners in order to find the most dangerous points and combinations. The result was the birth of dim-mak. He concealed the most effective techniques and point combinations in a series of movements, which later became known as t'ai chi. Interestingly, the ancient acupuncturists had a method of self-defense that involved attacking dangerous acupuncture points with needles, fans, and brushes.[1] Because Zhang Sanfeng was also an acupuncturist, it is conceivable that dim-mak could have evolved from this art.

Some believe that Zhang Sanfeng was actually a student of a man named Feng Yiyuan. In another theory of dim-mak's origin, Feng Yiyuan is credited with creating a system of attacking 36 of the most dangerous acupuncture points. Feng Yiyuan's students are believed to have first increased the number of points to 72 and then, later, to 108. According to this theory, Yiyuan's system eventually surfaced at the Southern Shaolin Temple and became integrated into many different styles.[2] Numerous martial arts have been influenced by or developed from those practiced at the Southern Shaolin Temple, which could explain why dim-mak is a component of so many traditional martial arts.

T'ai chi, eagle claw, monk fist, and white crane are just of few of the Chinese martial arts that involve attacking the dim-mak points. Evidence of the connection between dim-mak and Okinawan karate can be found in an old Okinawan manuscript called the *Bubishi*, which can be traced back to 17th-century China.[3] For hundreds of years, Okinawan masters have been passing this manuscript, which contains numerous descriptions of dim-mak, including point locations and the delayed death touch,[4] to their most advanced and trusted students. It is believed that the secrets of dim-mak were integrated into the traditional Okinawan katas. Okinawan karate eventually migrated to Japan and Korea. Comparing the Okinawan katas with those of the Japanese and Korean styles reveals their shared connection to dim-mak, as there are a number of similar movements.

In the past, the location of the points and methods of attacking them were only taught behind closed doors to the most advanced students. Often, only a single student was taught the true dim-mak interpretation of a form. Given the lethal effectiveness of such an art, it is understandable that the old masters felt a sense of responsibility and attempted to keep the art out of the wrong hands. However, this practice set the foundation for the growth of controversy. Because many "masters" learned only the movements of the forms and not the true dim-mak meanings hidden within them, dim-mak was withheld from generations of teachers and students. Thus, martial artists have been practicing an ineffective method of self-defense for many years, and as a result, the arts have lost much of their credibility. In being denied access to this information, many dedicated martial artists have been cheated. The time has come for all serious students to have the option of learning the truth behind their art, and that truth lies in the secret teachings of dim-mak.

As mentioned, dim-mak has resurfaced in recent years and is now being taught openly. There are martial artists who have discovered this knowledge and started teaching it publicly because they believe that all martial artists should have access to it. This has resulted in the open teaching of dim-mak by others who believe that if it is going to be available, it should be taught in its entirety to avoid the possibility of unintentional injury. Overall, this has had a positive impact on the martial arts, but there is still an issue of public safety that needs to be addressed. There are those who are repeatedly striking the dim-mak points in seminars and in practice in order to demonstrate that they work. Others are striking the points on students to see if they work. Still others believe that striking the points is harmless. The latter is far from the truth, and it is time that people were informed about the true dangers inherent in the practice of dim-mak. Even the simple "knockout" performed at many seminars is quite dangerous. Many of the techniques that cause a knockout actually cause a sudden drop in blood pressure, which generally results in fainting. However, medical research has shown that a sudden drop in blood pressure can cause myocardial ischemic events (i.e., the deprivation of oxygen to the heart muscle, which can lead to a heart attack) in a person with preexisting heart disease.[5] Given the overall prevalence of coronary heart disease in modern society, one could extrapolate that a number of people attending seminars could have some form of heart disease, and if one of them were "knocked out," he or she could suffer a heart attack. If you are not convinced already, as you read this book it should become evident that attacking the dim-mak points can adversely affect both the nervous and cardiovascular systems and that this is, in fact, very dangerous.

Since the ability to use the points in combat requires a great deal of skill and training, the danger of someone's learning the points for the sole purpose of causing harm is not a major concern. Most people of that mentality lack the discipline needed to develop such skills. The real danger lies in the application of such techniques by the skilled but uninformed martial artist. It is conceivable that a skilled, advanced student could utilize the points of dim-mak either in practice or on the street and thereby unintentionally cause great harm. Thus, anyone involved in learning dim-mak should have access to information about its medical dangers—and not necessarily in the form of ancient riddles or acupuncture theories. For many, the only credible information is that based on modern medical science.

At first glance, a physician writing a book about striking the nervous system through acupuncture points would seem to contradict the first principle of medicine—*primum nonnocere*: first do no harm. Why would a doctor write a book about such a dangerous martial art? The answer to this enigma is actually quite simple and lies in the philosophy of a unique form of medicine called osteopathic medicine.

Osteopathic medicine was created out of a need during the late 1800s. Medical science was in its infancy, and many of the medical treatments of the time were not very helpful and often hazardous. An American physician by the name of Andrew Taylor Still started to investigate alternative methods of healing after losing three of his children to meningitis. Even though he was a medical doctor, he was unable to do anything to save his children. This was before antibiotics, and the only medications available were toxic substances with a mercury base or narcotics. Bloodletting, which involves slicing open an artery and draining a person's blood, was still a widely practiced treatment. Following the death of his children, Dr. Still lost faith in such treatments and postulated that the human body must have an innate ability to heal itself. He spent a great deal of time researching and concluded that the proper functioning of the nervous system in combination with the unimpeded flow of blood and lymph was the secret to unleashing the body's ability to heal. Through his research, he discovered that the musculoskeletal system exerted a significant influence over the nervous, circulatory, and lymphatic systems. Based upon that research, he developed a system of musculoskeletal manipulative treatments that enhanced the function of these three systems. He called his new system of medicine osteopathy.[6]

It should be noted that this early version of osteopathic medicine migrated to many countries and remained static, while, in the United States, it continued to evolve as medical science advanced. This discrepancy in evolution has resulted in two different versions of osteopathic medicine. In the United States, an osteopathic physician is a licensed medical doctor with training in all modern methods of medical treatment plus additional training in osteopathic manipulation and philosophy. In those countries where the early version of osteopathic medicine did not evolve, osteopathic physicians are not medical doctors, and their training is limited to manipulation. This text will discuss the evolution of osteopathic medicine in the United States.

The curriculum at early osteopathic medical schools included manipulation, surgery, obstetrics, and gynecology. There was no training in pharmacology, and the early osteopathic doctors did not use medications. When antibiotics and other effective medications became available, the curriculum at the osteopathic medical schools changed to include pharmacology, and the use of medications became standard. Today, the curriculum at an osteopathic medical school is identical to that at an allopathic school (M.D. granting school), but it includes courses in osteopathic medicine as well. Thus, the osteopathic medical student receives an enormous amount of additional education in the nervous and musculoskeletal systems. It is this aspect of his or her education that gives the osteopathic physician a unique perspective on health and disease. This is also the reason the study of osteopathic medicine is especially suited to the study of the relationship between dim-mak and the nervous system.

Upon graduating, osteopathic physicians are awarded a D.O. (doctor of osteopathic medicine) degree, which identifies them as having specialized training. Many go on to train alongside their M.D. counterparts in the medical specialties such as internal medicine, surgery, cardiology, and so on. In the United States, there is no difference in the licensing of the D.O. and M.D. Both are considered medical doctors; however, the osteopathic physician has a different philosophy of medicine. Osteopathic medicine is a holistic form of modern medicine that considers the human body to be an integrated organism, and it considers the prevention of illness to be of the utmost importance. Within this emphasis on prevention lies the resolution to the enigma of a medical doctor's decision to write a book about dim-mak.

Today, it is very easy to find information on the techniques and points of dim-mak. One can choose from a number of books, videos, and seminars. Almost all of these sources explain dim-mak using the theories and nomenclature of acupuncture. Although there are many references on acupuncture theories, many people are unfamiliar with them or just do not understand them. The lack of a modern scientific explanation for dim-mak has led some martial artists to reject its ancient teachings and warnings as mystical nonsense and to question its effectiveness. Dangerous experimentation on students or unsuspecting victims is a very real consequence of such ignorance. Perhaps this can be avoided once knowledge of the dangers inherent in the practice of dim-mak is readily available from a credible source. It is hoped that the modern medical explanation of dim-mak that follows will give merit to the ancient warnings, improve the art's credibility, and provide a pathway for its refinement.

Chapter 1

Science or Science Fiction?

M any have seen the dubbed, low-budget martial arts movies that depict the martial arts master as having almost magical powers. The martial arts world is inundated with tales of ancient masters who could cause instant or delayed death or illness by attacking secret points. Many believe that such tales, although fascinating, are nothing more than fictional nonsense. When the ancient art of dim-mak resurfaced through the efforts of a few knowledgeable masters, many skeptics were forced to reconsider their position concerning the existence of such skills. Although many people have witnessed the devastating effects of dim-mak on videotapes and at seminars, there are still those who remain in doubt. This could be due to the fact that dim-mak is normally explained based on ancient theories of acupuncture and an internal energy called chi. The concept of chi, or ki, is alien to the Western mind, and thus the idea of attacking certain points to affect a person's energy flow seems ludicrous. Without seeing a clear connection between the points and the organs, it is difficult to accept that attacking a point can damage an internal organ. Furthermore, the paradoxical concept that the points can both injure and heal makes dim-mak even harder for the logical mind to comprehend. Thus, it is easy to understand why so many dismiss dim-mak as nothing more than mystical nonsense. However, when explained using modern medical science, dim-mak becomes less of a legend and more of a dangerous reality.

Dim-mak is based on the ancient art of acupuncture. According to acupuncture theory, there is a circulating life force that travels through distinct invisible pathways in the body. These pathways are called meridians, and each one is related to one of the internal organs. When the dim-mak points are attacked, it is believed that the flow of energy is disrupted, resulting in illness or death. The idea of a life force circulating through invisible channels is a difficult one for some of us to accept. However, when this life force is explained as electricity, the concept becomes much more reasonable to the Western mind. The dim-mak points are usually located very close to or directly on a nerve. Therefore, the manipulation of a point could easily stimulate the adjacent nerve. The nervous system works through minute electrical impulses. Any electrical current, no matter how diminutive, gives off electromagnetic radiation. Thus, one could conclude that the points are really doorways to the nervous system, and that the circulating life force is actually the electrical activity of the nervous system. Further evidence of the correlation between the acupuncture meridians and the nervous system can be seen in the phenomenon of referred pain. One especially important example involves the radiation of pain down the arm during a heart attack. The pain traveling down the arm is a direct result of stimulation of the ulnar nerve. This is easily explained by the neurological connection in the spinal cord between the ulnar nerve and the sympathetic nerves of the heart. However, the path of the pain down the arm also corresponds to the heart meridian in acupuncture. Is this just coincidence, or is it two explanations of the same phenomenon based on the perspectives of different cultures?

To some, the concept of attacking an internal organ by stimulating a point on the skin seems like a feat of magic. However, if one can accept the idea that a dim-mak point is an avenue for attacking the nervous system, then it becomes easier to understand how the points can affect the internal organs. There is an area of the body where the peripheral nerves connect with nerves from the internal organs. This connection is well known in neurology and is called convergence. Usually, by tracing the major nerve affected by a stimulated point, it is possible to find a neurological pathway leading directly to an internal organ. Furthermore, medical research has shown that stimulating the peripheral nerves can adversely affect the internal organs.[1] Thus, stimulating an external nerve through a dim-mak point can stimulate the nerves that are connected to the internal organs, resulting in damage. Once the pathway is mapped out by the neurological connections, the concept of attacking an internal organ through a dim-mak point seems much more plausible.

There is a theory in acupuncture called the five-element theory. In this theory, each meridian is assigned one of five elements: fire, metal, wood, earth, and water. The five-element theory describes the interrelationships of the meridians according to the cycle of destruction or the cycle of creation. The cycle of destruction states that fire will melt metal, metal will cut wood, wood will destroy earth, earth will destroy water, and water will destroy fire. This means that stimulation of a meridian will cause the inhibition of the meridian that follows it in the cycle of destruction. In dim-mak, the cycle of destruction is sometimes used to determine the sequence of the point attacks. For example, if one stimulated a fire point before a metal point, the effect on the metal point would be exaggerated because fire melts metal. This seemingly mystical ancient theory is supported by modern neuroscience. The points on the ulnar nerve, which are considered fire points, are located along the underside of the arm. The points on the radial nerve, which are considered metal points, are located along the top of the arm. If one stimulates the ulnar nerve prior to stimulating the radial nerve, the effect of the radial nerve attack is exaggerated. However, this effect does not work in reverse.

Although the five-element theory provides one explanation for this phenomenon, modern neuroscience provides another. When a nerve senses pain, it sends a signal to the spinal cord. This signal then travels up the spinal cord to the brain. The pain signal also travels up one or two segments of the spinal cord on a separate pathway. The segment of the spinal cord where the radial nerve enters is located higher than where the ulnar nerve enters. Thus, stimulation of the ulnar nerve can send a pain signal up to the segment where the radial nerve enters. As a result, when the radial nerve is stimulated, the segment receives pain signals from two separate sources. These pain signals then work synergistically to send an even greater pain signal to the brain. However, because pain usually travels *up* the spinal cord to the brain, the radial nerve cannot send a pain signal down to the level where the ulnar nerve enters. Consequently, striking the radial nerve before the ulnar nerve does not intensify the pain of the latter strike. Which is a better explanation, the five-element theory or neuroscience? It probably depends on one's culture and level of education.

One aspect of dim-mak that sounds as if it's straight out of a science fiction movie is that of death points. How can it be possible for a person to strike another person on specific areas of the body and thereby cause death? Such a concept evokes images of the Vulcan death grip. However, a number of medical journals contain case descriptions and studies of sudden death secondary to chest trauma. In one study, for instance, there was evidence that a fatal heart rhythm could be caused by trauma to a specific area of the chest.[2] Interestingly, the area of impact used in the study correlated with one of the "death points" described in dim-mak.

Discussion of the autonomic nervous system brings forth another interesting correlation between dim-mak and the nervous system. Dim-mak and acupuncture both involve theories that are based on the concept of yin and yang, which permeates all aspects of Eastern cultures. The yin and yang concept postulates that everything in the universe has an opposite. According to the theories of acupuncture and dim-mak, the meridians have either yin or yang properties. The yang meridians are related to the solid organs and are believed to have a positive energy. The yin meridians are related to the hollow organs and are believed to have a negative energy. The body is considered to be in a state of health when these two energies are in balance. Thus, in acupuncture, the effects of dim-mak are explained by an imbalance of yin and yang in the body. Interestingly, there is a correlation between the theory of yin and yang and modern neuroscience. The autonomic nervous system has two components, the parasympathetic and sympathetic nervous systems, which have opposing actions on the internal organs. One will speed up the functioning of an organ, and the other will slow it down. In other words, one will have a positive effect, and the other will have a negative effect. It is well known in Western medicine that an imbalance between the parasympathetic and sympathetic nervous systems can cause illness and even death. Recent research has shown that many cases of sudden cardiac death can be attributed to an imbalance in the autonomic nervous system.[3] Interestingly, stimulation of the dim-mak points can directly affect the balance of the autonomic nervous system. When the dim-mak points are attacked, is one causing an imbalance between yin and yang or an imbalance in the autonomic nervous system?

What about the subject of a delayed death touch? Could such a sinister method of attacking a human being be a reality? If the spleen were attacked through the left 8th and 9th ribs and the force was hard enough to fracture the ribs and tear the spleen, the answer would be yes. When the spleen is ruptured, the capsule around the spleen controls the bleeding for a short period of time. During this interval, the individual will have no symptoms. Eventually, the spleen capsule bursts and the individual bleeds to death almost instantly. This window of time without symptoms is well known to trauma surgeons. It is interesting that there is a legend of a three-day death touch and that the window of time mentioned can last three days.

How can there be points that have two different effects depending on how they are stimulated? Even if one accepts the notion that one is attacking the nervous system, it is still difficult to believe that a point can cause two different effects. The answer to this paradox lies in the study of neuroscience. The peripheral nerves are actually a bundle of multiple nerve fibers of different types. When a nerve is attacked, a certain type of nerve fiber called type C transmits a pain signal to the spinal cord. The stimulation of the type C nerve fibers causes severe pain that affects the autonomic nervous system. Massage or acupuncture stimulates a different type of nerve fiber called type A. This type of nerve fiber also carries a pain signal to the spinal cord. However, the pain associated with the type A nerve fiber is a sharp, well-localized pain that is relatively mild in comparison to that associated with the type C nerve fiber. In fact, an itch is caused by the stimulation of type A nerve fibers. Interestingly, stimulation of the type A nerve fibers has been shown to block the effects of the type C nerve fibers by inhibiting the type C nerve signal in the spinal cord. Thus, various methods of point stimulation can have different effects depending on the type of nerve fiber that is activated. This is also why the effects of attacking a point can be reversed with acupuncture or massage.

The subject of healing, or revival, brings forth another interesting aspect of dim-mak that is supported by medical science. When an opponent is "knocked out," he or she is revived either by slapping the trapezium or by pressing a point at the base of the skull. How can such methods be effective?

The slapping activates a nerve called the spinal accessory nerve. This nerve is connected to an area of the brain called the reticular activating system, which is normally responsible for arousing a person from sleep. When the spinal accessory nerve is stimulated with a slap, it stimulates the ascending reticular activating system, causing the person to wake up. Pressing the point at the base of the skull stimulates a nerve that can inhibit the effects of the autonomic nervous system and allow the system to "reset." The unconscious individual will wake up when the system reverts back to normal activity. Similarly, there is an area of the back that is believed to activate the heart after a cardiac arrest. This sounds like the most ludicrous myth of all. However, the dorsal nerve roots are located on the back along the sides of the spinal cord. These nerve roots have connections to the sympathetic nerves of the internal organs. The area that is stimulated to revive the heart correlates with the dorsal nerve roots that are connected to the heart. Stimulation of this area causes an increase in the activity of the sympathetic nerves connected to the heart. These nerves stimulate the heart by releasing a chemical called epinephrine, which can restore a heartbeat in someone who is in cardiac arrest. In fact, the current medical treatment for cardiac arrest involves an injection of epinephrine. It is fascinating how the slapping of points on the back can stimulate the heart just like an injection of a life-saving drug.

Attacking dim-mak points to cause physical harm is a very real and dangerous method of fighting that has been taught using ancient nomenclature based more on culture than science. This has resulted in legends of martial artists possessing supernatural powers. The true practitioner of this art is far from supernatural. More than likely, the practitioner is an advanced student of the martial arts who has used the ancient nomenclature as a means to an end because there was no alternative. This does not make the art any less of a reality. The effects of dim-mak are based on physiology and can be explained by modern medical science. Thus, medical

science provides the martial artist with an alternative explanation of dim-mak. What is truly amazing is how the ancient
masters were able to develop such a complex method of
attacking the human body based on a theory that evolved
from observation. As one becomes involved in unraveling the
mystery of dim-mak, the true genius of its founders becomes
brutally, and painfully, apparent.

Chapter 2

The Nervous System

There may be some esoteric components of the martial arts that are not explained by modern science. It could very well be that modern science has not matured enough to explain all aspects of dim-mak. However, many of dim-mak's effects can be explained by neuroscience and neurocardiology. Thus, it is essential for one to have a basic understanding of the nervous system in order to comprehend the medical science behind dim-mak. The material in this section can be quite complex and requires some exertion on the part of the reader, but it is well worth the effort. In this section, the nervous system will be broken down into its components and the basic physiology will be discussed. It is important for the reader to understand the basic aspects of the autonomic nervous system as well as certain terms like *facilitation, convergence,* and *aberrant reference* because many of the later chapters will build upon these concepts.

There are two basic components of the human nervous system: the central nervous system and the peripheral nervous system. The central nervous system is composed of the brain and spinal cord. The peripheral nervous system consists of all the other nerves in the body. The peripheral nervous system is further divided into the somatic and autonomic nervous systems. (See Figure 1.)

The somatic nervous system is composed of the motor nerves that control the muscles and the sensory nerves monitoring pain, temperature, and position. Most of the dim-mak points are located on the peripheral nerves of the somatic system. Thus, for the remainder of this book, references to the peripheral nervous system will imply the peripheral somatic nerves. Attacking points located on the motor nerves can cause pain and paralysis. Attacking points located on the sensory nerves can cause severe pain. In addition, the somatic nervous system has neurological connections to the autonomic nerves of the internal organs. This is significant because stimulation of the somatic nervous system can produce changes in the autonomic nervous system.[1] This is the neurological link between the dim-mak points and the autonomic nervous system.

Most of dim-mak's effects, including knockout, heart attack, and cardiac arrest, can be explained by changes in

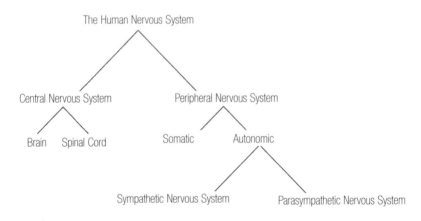

FIGURE 1
Breakdown of the nervous system.

the autonomic nervous system. This system unconsciously controls blood pressure, heart rate, digestion, urination, defecation, sleep, and breathing. The two components of this system, the sympathetic and the parasympathetic nervous systems, act on the internal organs in an antagonistic manner. One increases the activity of an organ and the other decreases the activity of the same organ. Some of the organs, such as the stomach and intestines, are stimulated by the parasympathetic nervous system. Other organs, such as the heart and lungs, are stimulated by the sympathetic nervous system. At this point, it is not important to know the effects of each system on each organ. The important concept is that each organ is affected by both of these systems in a different manner.

In summary, the nervous system is composed of the central and the peripheral nervous systems. The central nervous system consists of the brain and spinal cord. The peripheral nervous system is composed of all the other nerves, including the autonomic nervous system. One should think of autonomic as automatic because this component of the nervous system controls many functions of the body (including blood pressure, heart rate, respiration, digestion, and waste elimination) without any conscious input from the brain. The autonomic nervous system is further divided into the sympathetic and parasympathetic nervous systems and is responsible for most of dim-mak's effects.

SYMPATHETIC NERVOUS
SYSTEM AND CONVERGENCE

Anytime a person feels nervous, he or she is experiencing the effects of the sympathetic nervous system. The sympathetic nervous system is an ancient component of man's evolution that has a very important survival function. Stimulation of this the part of the nervous system results in that apprehensive, queasy feeling one experiences when under stress or in danger. This feeling is part of the fight or flight response, so named because it prepares us to either engage in battle or run from danger. When the sympathetic nervous system is stimulated, the heart rate increases, blood pressure rises, blood flow to the muscles increases, blood glucose increases, and the digestive organs shut down. All of these effects occur unconsciously and automatically. When excessively stimulated, the sympathetic nervous system can cause constipation, anxiety, and even death due to its effects on the heart.

Nerves from the sympathetic nervous system innervate

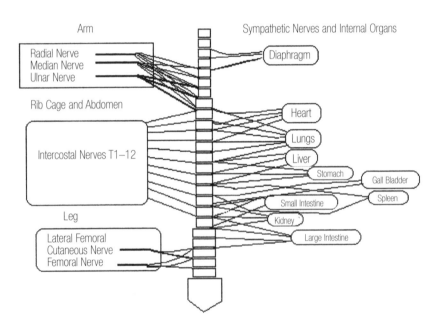

FIGURE 2
The left side of the diagram illustrates the peripheral nerves and their connections to the spinal cord. The right side of the diagram illustrates the levels where the sympathetic nerves from the internal organs connect to the spinal cord. As one can see, there are levels of the spinal cord where the peripheral and sympathetic nerves converge.

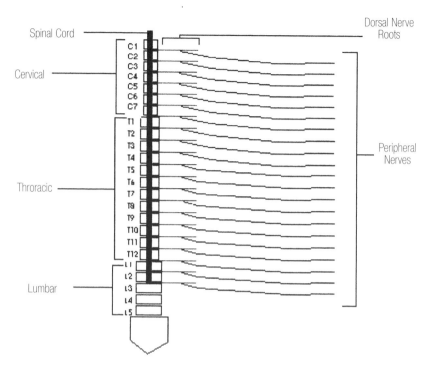

FIGURE 3
The short lines represent the spinal nerve roots and their connections to the sympathetic nerves of the internal organs. The longer lines represent the peripheral nerves. This diagram illustrates the connection between the sympathetic nerves and the peripheral nerves just before both enter the spinal cord.

each organ. The sympathetic nerves of the internal organs connect directly to the spinal cord and have a dual purpose. They supply sympathetic stimulation and sense pain in the internal organs. This is important because these nerves fuse with external nerves that are vulnerable through dim-mak points. (See Figures 2 and 3.) This fusion of external nerves and internal organ sympathetic nerves is called convergence. The actual connections occur in the dorsal nerve roots, which are located under the bladder points next to the spine (see fig. 4).

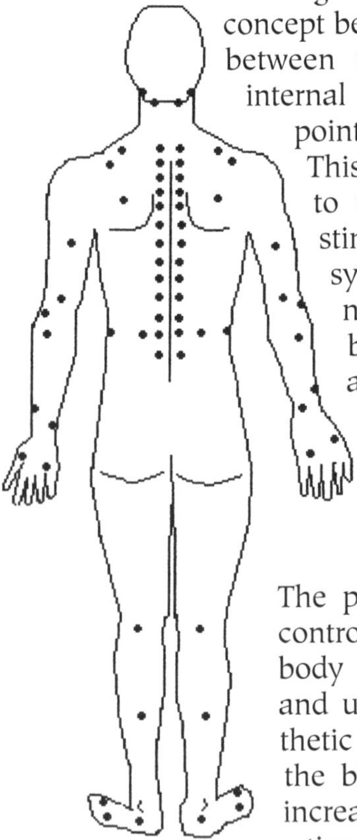

Convergence is an extremely important concept because it is the neurological link between the dim-mak points and the internal organs. Attacking a dim-mak point stimulates the external nerve. This stimulation can be propagated to the dorsal nerve root causing stimulation of the internal organ sympathetic nerves. Since these nerves also monitor pain, the brain perceives such stimulation as pain coming from one of the internal organs.

PARASYMPATHETIC NERVOUS SYSTEM

The parasympathetic nervous system controls the resting functions of the body such as digestion, defecation, and urination. When the parasympathetic nervous system is stimulated, the blood flow to the digestive tract increases, as does the process of digestion. The heart rate, blood pressure, and breathing slow down. All of these functions allow the individual to rest and replenish the cells of the body. Excessive stimulation of the parasympathetic nervous system can cause abdominal cramps, diarrhea, vomiting, knockout, and cardiac arrest. The parasympathetic nervous system is also responsible for many of dim-mak's effects, including the pressure point knockouts.

The parasympathetic nervous system consists of and is attacked through the cranial and sacral nerves.

All of the cranial nerves, which connect directly to the

FIGURE 4
Dim-mak points on the back of the body.

brain through the skull (cranium), are very effective at causing a knockout and can be attacked through points on the face and neck. All but one of the cranial nerves innervate the face, head, and neck. The major cranial nerve responsible for the parasympathetic stimulation of the internal organs is the vagus nerve. The vagus, trigeminal, and facial nerves are the three most important cranial nerves. The points on these nerves and their branches enable the martial artist to directly stimulate the parasympathetic nervous system. The vagus nerve transverses down the neck into the thoracic cavity, where it connects to the heart, lungs, and digestive system. Stimulation of this nerve directly increases the parasympathetic effects on these organs. The trigeminal nerve has three branches that correspond to most of the points on the face. The facial nerve also corresponds to many of the points on the face. There are other cranial nerves, but these three are the most affected by dim-mak and have the largest impact on the parasympathetic nervous system.

The genitals are also innervated by the parasympathetic nervous system through the sacral nerves. Consequently, striking the genitals can also stimulate the parasympathetic nervous system.

The main concept to appreciate is that stimulation of the cranial or genital nerves can directly stimulate the parasympathetic nervous system. The results of excessive parasympathetic stimulation include nausea, vomiting, diarrhea, abdominal cramps, knockout, and cardiac arrest. Such effects are directly dependent on the amount of parasympathetic stimulation. Diarrhea can result when the parasympathetic system increases the activity of the digestive tract. A knockout can result when the parasympathetic nervous system causes a sudden drop in blood pressure. Cardiac arrest can result when very strong parasympathetic activity slows the heart down until it comes to a complete stop.

SEGMENTATION

Segmentation is an important concept to understand because the dim-mak points are located on nerves that enter the spinal cord at very distinct levels. When these nerves are stimulated, they can affect the internal organs that are connected to the spinal cord at the same level because of convergence. For example, a strike to the Stomach 18 point will stimulate the fifth intercostal nerve. This nerve connects to the spinal cord at the level of the fifth thoracic vertebrae. This level is also neurologically connected to the heart. Thus, the heart could be affected by stimulation of the fifth intercostal nerve. Through *segmentation* it is possible to trace the neurologic connections between the dim-mak points and the internal organs.

Each segment of the spinal cord and spine is connected to different internal organs and nerves. Each segment consists of a vertebra and a portion of the spinal cord, and each innervates different areas of the body. The specific area that is innervated by a given segment is called a dermatome. All of the points in a specific dermatome will affect the same spinal level and the same internal organ. Consequently, knowledge of the dermatomes allows one to determine which internal organ will be affected by a dim-mak point or combination. This sectioning of the spinal cord according to the number of vertebrae and dermatomes is known in neurology as segmentation.

The spinal cord is divided into twenty-four vertebrae and five fused sacral segments (see fig. 5). It is further divided into seven cervical, twelve thoracic, and five lumbar vertebrae. The cervical vertebrae are usually designated with a capital C and a number from 1 to 7 corresponding to the level of the spinal cord. For example, C7 is the seventh cervical vertebrae from the base of the skull. There are eight cervical nerves, the first of which exits the spine above C1 and the last of which exits below C7. The thoracic vertebrae are labeled with a capital T

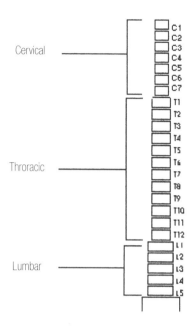

FIGURE 5
Segmentation of spinal cord.

and a number from 1 to 12. For example, T5 is the fifth thoracic vertebrae down from C7. There are twelve thoracic nerve roots, and each one exits the spine below the vertebrae. The lumbar vertebrae are labeled with a capital L and a number from 1 to 5. Like the thoracic nerves, the lumbar nerves exit the spine below each vertebra. The sacrum is the fusion of five bones at the end of the spine. The pelvic parasympathetic nerves are located in this area. These nerves innervate the genitals and part of the large intestine.

The dorsal nerve roots are located along the levels of the thoracic vertebrae and the first two lumbar vertebrae. The dorsal nerve root is where the sympathetic nerves, the intercostal nerves, and the external nerves fuse. There are 14 dorsal nerve roots located in the area from T1 to L2 (see figs. 3 and 4). Each internal organ has a distinct level where its sympathetic nerves connect to the spinal cord and dorsal nerve roots (see Table 1). For example, the heart has sympathetic nerves that enter the spinal cord along the first five thoracic vertebrae.

TABLE 1:
THE SPINAL LEVEL OF ORGAN
AND LIMB SYMPATHETIC INNERVATION

Organ	Spinal Level
Heart	T1–5 bilateral
Lungs	T1–4 bilateral
Stomach	T6–9 on left
Gall Bladder	T6 on right
Spleen	T7 on left
Pancreas	T7 on right
Liver	T5 on right
Kidney	T10–11 bilateral
Small Intestine	T10–11 bilateral
Colon	T10–L2
Arms	T2–8
Legs	T11–L2

REFLEXES

The human body has an integrated network of reflexes that control everything from digestion and blood pressure to the avoidance of pain. Reflexes can explain many aspects of dim-mak. Some reflexes, like the ones that regulate digestion, respiration, blood pressure, and heartbeat, occur unconsciously through the autonomic nervous system. These can be exploited by attacking the dim-mak points, which can result in fainting, digestive disturbances, and even death. In addition, the manipulation of reflexes can enable us to use an opponent's strength to our advantage.

Unconscious reflexes will cause a person to move away from pain and are important in the application of medical science to dim-mak. This is especially true regarding the grappling methods of dim-mak. The withdrawal reflex is one that many have experienced. This reflex occurs in response to pain and serves to minimize the damage that would result if the body part were not moved. The classic example is when a person touches something very hot like a burning stove and the hand is unconsciously pulled away from the heat.

The withdrawal reflex can actually occur in any direction. Pain in the sole of the foot, such as when stepping on a tack, will cause the foot to come up. Pain in the back will cause a person to move forward. Pain in the abdomen will cause a person to bend forward. As can be seen, it does not matter were the pain enters. When a nerve is stimulated, the body will move instinctively to minimize the pain and damage. Thus, when familiar with the patterns of these reflexes, one can use them to manipulate an opponent. For example, to move an opponent in a given direction while grappling, all one has to do is cause pain in a nerve opposite that direction by attacking a dim-mak point. The opponent's body will move in the desired direction reflexively.

Also important in the application of medical science to dim-mak is the crossed extensor reflex. This may seem complicated but is actually part of the withdrawal reflex. When a stimulus causes pain in a limb, the limb will be withdrawn from the stimulus and the opposite limb will extend to facilitate pushing the stimulus away. To understand how this applies to all four limbs, think of a cat stepping on a tack. If the right front paw stepped on the tack, the left front leg and right rear leg would straighten so the cat could pull the injured front right paw up while still maintaining its balance. The martial artist can exploit this same principle while grappling. For example, if one were to attack a dim-mak point on an opponent's lower leg or foot, the crossed extensor reflex would cause his same-side arm to straighten. As a result, the joints of the arm and shoulder would be vulnerable to hyper-extension or an arm lock.

Reflexes also affect muscle strength. This can be used in the manipulation of joints. Painful stimulation of a nerve results in a loss of power in the muscle it innervates. This is called reflex paralysis. When there is a decrease in the strength of a muscle supporting a joint, the joint is vulnerable to dislocation. Thus, a martial artist could use reflex paralysis to weaken a joint so that he can dislocate it with a follow-up technique.

Perhaps the most important reflexes are those concerning the autonomic nervous system. The parasympathetic mediated reflexes can be manipulated to induce fainting or cardiac arrest. The sympathetic mediated reflexes can be manipulated to induce a fatal arrhythmia (irregular heart rhythm), to cause pain in an internal organ, or to enhance the parasympathetic reflexes. One particular reflex that bears mentioning here is the somatosympathetic reflex, which increases the activity of the sympathetic nervous system in response to pain. Thus, whenever the dim-mak points cause pain, they also cause an increase in the activity of the sympathetic nervous system. This reflex will become more important in later chapters, when dim-mak's effects on the heart are explained.

Somatovisceral Reflexes

Stimulation of the peripheral nervous system can cause a number of reflex changes in the internal organs known as somatovisceral reflexes.[2] For instance, it has been found that peripheral nerve stimulation can cause a decrease in the blood perfusion of the internal organs.[3] This can lead to severe organ damage, especially if the heart and kidneys are involved. In addition, stimulation of the peripheral nervous system has also been found to damage the internal organs directly.[4] Thus, since many of the dim-mak points are located on the peripheral nerves, the martial artist can exploit somatovisceral reflexes to damage the internal organs.

The original research on somatovisceral reflexes demonstrated that they would occur in response to mechanical stimulation of the peripheral nerves, such as pinches and other quick, forceful movements. An electrical current failed to produce consistent results.[5] This is interesting because the same type of nerve stimulation occurs when the dim-mak points are attacked by a quick, forceful strike or grasp. Thus, attacking the dim-mak points can cause somatovisceral reflexes.

Somatovisceral reflexes are important for a number of reasons. First, the research behind them provides evidence that the dim-mak points can affect the internal organs. If there is scientific evidence that peripheral nerve stimulation can damage the internal organs, then there is scientific evidence that the dim-mak points can damage the internal organs because the dim-mak points can cause peripheral nerve stimulation. Second, stimulation of a given nerve will only cause a somatovisceral reflex in the internal organs connected to the same section of the spinal cord. Thus, by knowing the segmentation of the nervous system one can predict which internal organ will be affected by a dim-mak point or combination.

SUMMATION

Summation is a neurological term that describes how the stimulation of a nerve can be enhanced by stimulation of additional nerves that affect the same section of the spinal cord or brain. To clarify, when two or more nerves that connect to the same section of the spinal cord are stimulated, the effect of the stimulation on the spinal cord is greater. This can be translated into use for dim-mak by realizing that the effects of attacking a nerve can be magnified by the stimulation of another nerve with similar effects. For example, the cranial nerves and the carotid sinus can both increase the activity of the parasympathetic nervous system. The concept of summation means that if one attacked either multiple cranial nerves or a combination of cranial nerves and the carotid sinus there would be a greater increase in the activity of the parasympathetic nervous system. Thus, stimulation of the parasympathetic nervous system by multiple methods will have a synergistic effect. Conversely, stimulation of the sympathetic nervous system by multiple methods will also have a synergistic effect.

This concept can also be applied to the different methods of attacking the internal organs. Attacking certain peripheral nerves can cause a somatovisceral reflex affecting an internal organ. Thus, stimulating multiple nerves that all affect the same spinal level magnifies the effect on the internal organ. For example, attacking multiple points connected to the spinal cord at T6–9 would enhance the effect on the stomach (refer to Table 1). If a strike to the stomach occurred at the same time, the effect would be even more devastating.

In summary, the concept of summation means that the effects of attacking a nerve can be increased by simultaneously attacking other nerves that have similar effects. This can be applied to effects on the sympathetic nervous system, the parasympathetic nervous system, or a specific spinal level and internal organ.

FACILITATION

Facilitation is a neurological term that describes the sensitization of the spinal cord at a specific level. When a nerve is struck through a dim-mak point, it sends a barrage of pain signals to the spinal cord. This causes the other nerves that connect at the same spinal level to become hyperresponsive. In other words, the subsequent attack will have greater effects because the spinal cord was prestimulated by the initial strike. The major difference between summation and facilitation is that the latter does not involve simultaneous stimulation of the nerves.

A facilitated spinal segment can also cause unstimulated nerves to be stimulated. This means that the spinal cord can actually stimulate the nerves to which it is connected. This includes the sympathetic nerves connected to the internal organs. If a facilitated spinal segment stimulated the sympathetic nerves of an internal organ, it could induce a somatovisceral reflex. There must be very strong pain signals entering the spinal cord for this to occur. The convergence between the sympathetic nerves of the internal organs and the peripheral nerves occurs in areas of the spinal cord called the fourth and fifth laminae. When the external nerves send multiple pain signals to these areas, the nerve cells in the spinal cord increase their rate of firing until a state of continuous discharge is attained.[6] This continuous activity of the spinal cord is responsible for stimulating the other nerves connected to the same level, especially the sympathetic nerves of the internal organs.

Facilitation can be applied to any area of the spine. One only needs to understand the concept and the affected spinal cord levels of the points used. For example, stimulation of one Stomach 18 point would cause the other Stomach 18 point to become hypersensitive. This occurs because the T5 level of the spinal cord is facilitated by the attack to the first point. Consequently, any point connected to the T5 level of the spinal cord will be hypersensitive, including the other Stomach 18 point.

In another example, both the ulnar and radial nerves have branches that enter the spinal cord at the C7, C8, and T1 levels. If the ulnar nerve is struck before the radial nerve, the T1 segment will start getting a neurological stimulus from the ulnar strike. When the radial nerve is struck, the signal to the spinal cord at T1 is amplified because the ulnar nerve facilitated this level.

The third example involves the radial and phrenic nerves. The phrenic nerve controls the diaphragm and enters the spinal cord at the C3–5 level. This nerve is directly accessible under the Large Intestine 17 point. When this point is attacked, it can cause the diaphragm to go into a spasm, which makes the recipient of the strike feel as if he cannot breathe. The phrenic nerve becomes more vulnerable after the lung or large intestine points on the radial nerve are stimulated because both the radial and phrenic nerves have a root that connects to the spinal cord at C5. Thus, stimulation of the radial nerve through the lung and large intestine points causes the C5 level to become facilitated, which magnifies the effect of an attack to the phrenic nerve under Large Intestine 17.

Facilitation can also explain how some points can affect different organs depending on how they are set up. Many of the points are located on nerves that connect to the spinal cord at more than one level. These points can simultaneously stimulate multiple levels of the spinal cord. However, when one of the levels is facilitated, the effect is greatest at that level. For example, attacking the heart points on the arm facilitates the spinal cord levels connected to the heart. This causes all of the points connected to the T1–5 levels of the spinal cord to affect the heart. If the lung and large intestine points are attacked, the level of the spinal cord connected to the lungs is facilitated, which causes all the points connected to the T1–4 levels to affect the lungs. Any internal organ can be attacked in this manner if one understands the principles of convergence, segmentation, and facilitation.

ABERRANT REFERENCE

Aberrant reference is a key neurological concept with regard to the medical science behind the effects of dim-mak because it explains how the dim-mak points affect the internal organs when used in combination. It also helps to explain the effect of a dim-mak combination on a specific area of the body that is distant from the attacked points. Aberrant reference can cause facilitation of a spinal level, a somatovisceral reflex, or increased activity of the parasympathetic nervous system. Furthermore, since an aberrant reference combination increases the effects of the parasympathetic nervous system, it can cause a knockout or cardiac arrest.

In order to understand aberrant reference, one must first understand the concept of referred pain—that is, the manifestation of pain in a site distant from its origin. Referred pain can be explained by the neurological connections in the spinal cord between the peripheral nerves and the internal organ sympathetic nerves. The pain from a diseased or injured organ is sensed by the sympathetic nerves and communicated to the spinal cord. Consequently, the convergence between the sympathetic and peripheral nerves enables pain from the internal organs to be propagated to the peripheral nerves. The result is that a person can feel pain from an internal organ in a completely different area of the body. For example, the pain from a heart attack may travel down either arm, up to the jaw, or even to the back.

Aberrant reference is a neurological term used to describe the displacement of referred pain. It is caused by simultaneous pain in two or more areas of the body. Neurologists have found that when a person is suffering with pain in multiple areas, the pain can be displaced to somewhere in the middle.[7] For example, the pain from a heart attack is usually located in the chest. However, when a person has concomitant painful gall bladder disease, the pain is referred to the stomach. This is because the stomach sympathetic nerves enter the spinal cord at a level that is between the spinal cord connections of the heart and gall bladder (see fig. 6).

However, it is not the location of the organs but rather the levels of the spinal cord that they are connected to that causes the displacement of pain. Aberrant reference is caused by pain signals entering the spinal cord at two or more levels. The pain is felt in the middle of where the multiple pain signals enter the spinal cord. In the preceding example, the stomach is innervated by nerves that connect to the spinal cord at the level of T6–7. This is directly in the middle of where the heart (T1–5) and the gall bladder (T7–8) connect to the spinal cord.

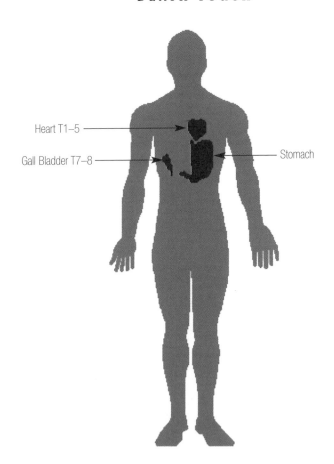

Heart T1–5

Gall Bladder T7–8

Stomach

FIGURE 6
The stomach connects to the spinal cord at the level of T6-7. Thus,
the pain from a heart attack in combination with the pain from gall
bladder disease will cause pain in the stomach because it connects
to the spinal cord at a level that is directly in the middle of where
the two injured organs connect to the spinal cord.

In the same way, when multiple nerves are simultaneously stimulated through dim-mak points, the pain is felt in between the nerves. Put more simply, when multiple points are attacked, the body experiences pain somewhere in the middle of the points. Thus, simultaneously attacking multiple points can cause pain that seems to be coming from one of the internal organs. For example, a simultaneous attack to the Heart 3 point on the ulnar nerve (T1) and the Spleen 6 point on the tibial nerve (L4) can cause pain in the small intestine (T10).

Different organs can be affected depending on which nerves are attacked. For example, if one were to strike a point on the ulnar nerve (heart points), it would register mostly at T1. If this were simultaneous with an attack to the femoral nerve (L3), the pain would register at T7, which is in the middle of T1 and L3. Since this level of the spinal cord is connected to the sympathetic nerves of the stomach and gall bladder, the brain would interpret the attack as pain in either the stomach or gall bladder. (See Figures 7 and 8.)

If all of the points attacked were on the left side of the body, the pain would be in the stomach. Conversely, if all of the points attacked were on the right side of the body, the pain would be in the gall bladder. This is because some internal organs have more nerve fibers entering the spinal cord on

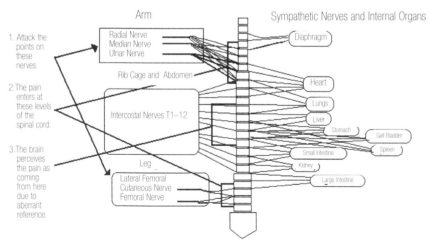

FIGURE 7
Aberrant reference.

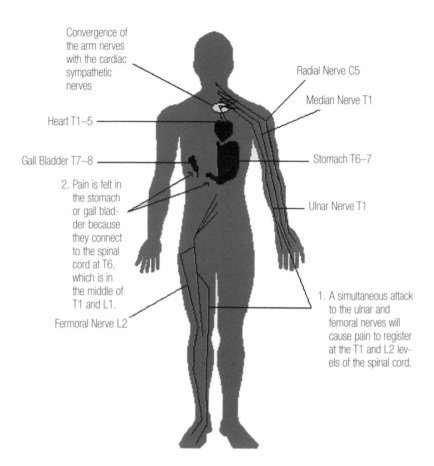

Convergence of
the arm nerves
with the cardiac
sympathetic
nerves

Radial Nerve C5

Median Nerve T1

Heart T1–5

Gall Bladder T7–8

Stomach T6–7

2. Pain is felt in
the stomach
or gall blad-
der because
they connect
to the spinal
cord at T6,
which is in
the middle of
T1 and L1.

Ulnar Nerve T1

Fermoral Nerve L2

1. A simultaneous attack
to the ulnar and
femoral nerves will
cause pain to register
at the T1 and L2 lev-
els of the spinal cord.

FIGURE 8
Example of aberrant reference.

one side. Examples include the liver, spleen, gall bladder, and
stomach. When multiple nerves on one side of the body are
stimulated, aberrant reference dictates that the pain will be
displaced to the internal organ located between the stimulated spinal levels on the same side. Since the gall bladder has
more sympathetic nerves entering the spinal cord on the right
side, stimulation of ulnar (T1) and femoral (L3) nerves on the

right will cause the pain to be felt in the gall bladder (T7). The opposite is true of the stomach because it has more sympathetic nerves entering the spinal cord on the left. Thus, stimulation of the same points on the left side will affect the stomach because its sympathetic nerves connect to the spinal cord at the same level (T7) but on the left side.

When nerves on the opposite arm and leg are attacked, the pain is displaced to the side with greater stimulation. A bilateral attack to points neurologically connected to the same spinal level will cause pain to register directly in the middle of the points. When this midway point corresponds to an internal organ, the pain will seem to be coming from that organ. For example, if one attacked the Stomach 18 point bilaterally (i.e., on both sides of the chest), the pain would stimulate the fifth intercostal nerves and be perceived as coming from the heart.

Because the intercostal nerves connect to the spinal cord at the same level as many of the internal organs, it is possible to use the arm or leg points to move the effect of an intercostal nerve strike either up or down. For example, attacking the Liver 13 point can cause a pain signal to enter the spinal cord along the 10th intercostal nerve (T10). If the lung points on the radial nerve (C5) were attacked at the same time, the pain would be displaced to the T1–2 level. Thus, a combination point strike affecting the radial and the tenth intercostal nerves can cause pain in the lungs. Similarly, a simultaneous strike to the Liver 13 point (T10) and the Liver 11 point (L2) can displace the pain to the T12–L1 level. Since the large intestine sympathetic nerves connect to the spinal cord at this level, the pain would be felt in the large intestine.

Many of the spinal levels can affect multiple organs. This can cause some confusion when attempting to pinpoint the internal organ affected by multiple points. This is where the concept of facilitation becomes important. The T1–4 levels of the spinal cord can affect either the heart or lungs. Which organ is affected depends on whether it's the heart points or the lung points that are attacked either prior to or during the aberrant reference technique. If the heart points are stimulated, they cause the T1–4 levels to affect the heart. Conversely, if the lung points are stimulated, they cause the T1–4 levels to affect the lungs.

A vasovagal faint (knockout) can be caused by severe pain in the heart, lungs, digestive tract, bladder, or genitals. Thus, one could cause a knockout by using the concept of aberrant reference to attack these internal organs. Because this will cause facilitation of a specific spinal level, it can also cause a somatovisceral reflex leading to organ dysfunction or failure. Aberrant reference combinations are synergistic with any other nerve that can cause increased parasympathetic effects or any other nerve that can cause a somatovisceral reflex affecting the same organ.

The concept of aberrant reference makes it possible to predict how combinations of dim-mak points will affect the body. This is important, because the areas affected are not always what one would expect. It also explains many of the effects of dim-mak including the reason attacking multiple points on the arms and legs can cause a knockout, illness, or death. The effects of both convergence and aberrant reference on the sympathetic nerves of the internal organs provide explanations for dim-mak's effects on the internal organs. Additionally, the concept of aberrant reference is useful when attempting to find synergistic point combinations. (This will become very helpful in later chapters.)

THE SYNAPSE

There are many different nerves in the human nervous system, and they communicate with each other through synapses, which are microscopic gaps between the nerves. The synapse is important because it is an area where a nerve signal can be enhanced or inhibited. When an impulse gets to the end of a nerve axon (the long portion of the nerve cell), it stimulates the release of chemicals called neurotransmitters, which then diffuse across the tiny gap and cause either stimulation or inhibition of the adjacent nerve. When an excitatory neurotransmitter is secreted, the adjacent nerve will be stimulated, and when an inhibitory neurotransmitter is secreted, the adjacent nerve will be inhibited. There are areas where multiple nerves will synapse with the same nerve. Stimulation of these nerves can prestimulate the adjacent nerve so that it becomes hypersensitive and can therefore be activated with minimal stimulation. This is what occurs during facilitation, summation, and convergence.

The action of inhibitory neurotransmitters explains how it is possible to block the effects of an attack to certain points. There is a training method called iron shirt training that enables one to withstand a dim-mak attack with minimal effects. This skill is often attributed to the ability to focus internal energy in the area of the attacked point. Medical science may have an alternative explanation, however. The area of the brain that is responsible for causing a pressure point knockout is neurologically connected to the cortex, which is the area responsible for conscious thoughts. It is conceivable, then, that one could block a pressure point knockout by causing the cortex to release inhibitory neurotransmitters in certain areas of the brain. In addition, certain areas of the spinal cord (which are also connected to the cortex) can, when stimulated, block the transmission of pain by inhibiting the pain fibers in the spinal cord. This neurological connection between the spinal cord and the cortex makes it possible to block pain by learning to stimulate the areas that inhibit the pain signal in the spinal cord. Thus, iron shirt training may have more to do with training the cortex than controlling internal energy.

The purpose of this chapter was to establish a foundation in the basic aspects of neurology that relate to dim-mak. At this point, the reader should be familiar with the basic components of the human nervous system, including the central and peripheral nervous systems, the somatic and autonomic nervous systems, and the sympathetic and parasympathetic nervous systems. In addition, the convergence between the internal organ sympathetic nerves and the external nerves should be well understood because it will be referred to extensively throughout this book. An understanding of how the nervous system is segmented will also be essential when concepts such as aberrant reference, summation, and facilitation are applied to dim-mak in later chapters. Finally, the reader will need to be familiar with reflexes, particularly the somato-visceral reflexes, which will be discussed extensively in the chapter on attacking the internal organs. Although some of these concepts will be reiterated in the later chapters for the sake of clarity, from this point on it will be assumed that the reader has basic understanding of the definitions and concepts covered in this chapter.

Chapter 3

The Points

The vulnerable areas of the body that are exploited in the martial arts have many names, including dim-mak points, vital points, kyusho points, and pressure points. Because the original art that attacked the acupuncture points was called dim-mak, this book will refer to these areas as dim-mak points. The connection between these points and the nervous system lies in the definition of what a point actually is. Originally, these points were defined as areas where one could attack an opponent's internal energy. Such a concept is difficult to prove or explain in scientific terms. However, it is easy to prove that these points affect the nervous system. The dim-mak points are usually located on a vulnerable nerve, and in fact it is impossible to attack a point without attacking a nerve. The fact that the points are painful when attacked provides further evidence of their effect on the nervous system. Medical science has found that pain is sensed and conveyed to the brain through the nervous system; however, there is no scientific evidence that the acupuncture meridians can sense pain. Therefore, a dim-mak point can be defined scientifically as an area where one can directly stimulate the nervous system.

All of the nerves discussed in this book can be attacked through dim-mak points, which have been labeled using the nomenclature of acupuncture (see figs. 9–12) in order to simplify finding them. Some of the points are grouped according to their effects on the heart, and new terms for such groups are introduced here for the purpose of identification. Furthermore, since every nerve has numerous branches with different names, for the sake of simplicity only the major nerve that is affected by attacking the associated dim-mak point will be identified in this book. Occasionally, the points are actually located on a branch of the nerve that is mentioned; however, if each and every one of these branches were named, the continuity of the information would be compromised.

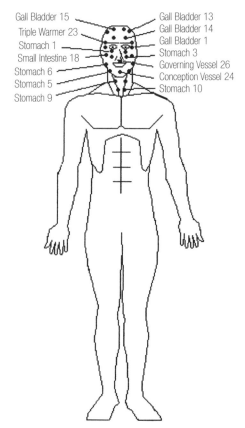

FIGURE 9
Above and Right: Head and neck points.

4 2

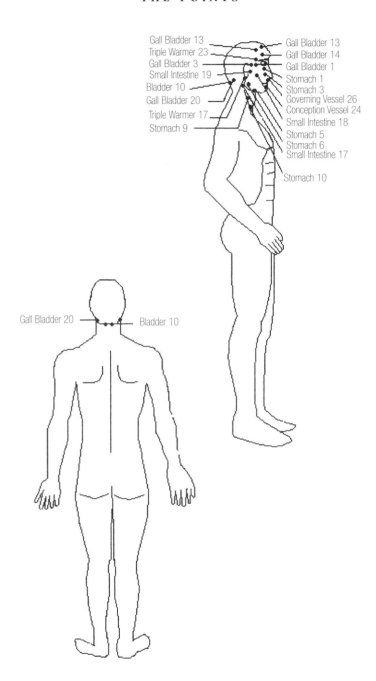

Gall Bladder 13
Triple Warmer 23
Gall Bladder 3
Small Intestine 19
Bladder 10
Gall Bladder 20
Triple Warmer 17
Stomach 9

Gall Bladder 13
Gall Bladder 14
Gall Bladder 1
Stomach 1
Stomach 3
Governing Vessel 26
Conception Vessel 24
Small Intestine 18
Stomach 5
Stomach 6
Small Intestine 17

Stomach 10

Gall Bladder 20

Bladder 10

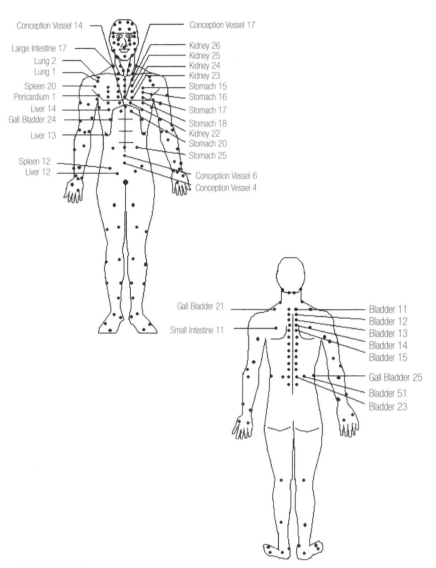

FIGURE 10
Points on the back and abdomen.

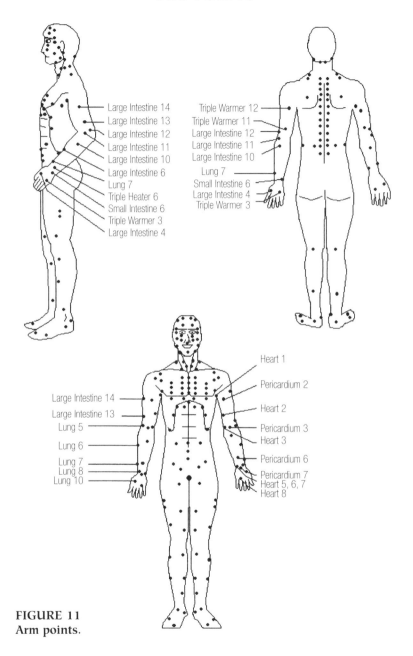

Large Intestine 14
Large Intestine 13
Large Intestine 12
Large Intestine 11
Large Intestine 10
Large Intestine 6
Lung 7
Triple Heater 6
Small Intestine 6
Triple Warmer 3
Large Intestine 4

Triple Warmer 12
Triple Warmer 11
Large Intestine 12
Large Intestine 11
Large Intestine 10
Lung 7
Small Intestine 6
Large Intestine 4
Triple Warmer 3

Heart 1
Pericardium 2
Heart 2
Pericardium 3
Heart 3
Pericardium 6
Pericardium 7
Heart 5, 6, 7
Heart 8

Large Intestine 14
Large Intestine 13
Lung 5
Lung 6
Lung 7
Lung 8
Lung 10

FIGURE 11
Arm points.

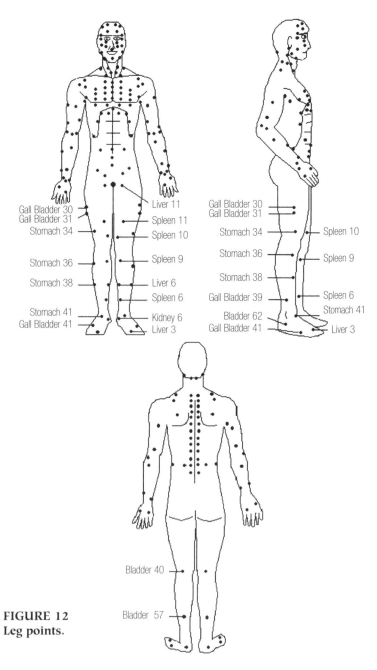

Gall Bladder 30
Gall Bladder 31
Stomach 34

Stomach 36

Stomach 38

Stomach 41
Gall Bladder 41

Liver 11
Spleen 11
Spleen 10

Spleen 9

Liver 6
Spleen 6

Kidney 6
Liver 3

Gall Bladder 30
Gall Bladder 31

Stomach 34

Stomach 36

Stomach 38

Gall Bladder 39

Bladder 62
Gall Bladder 41

Spleen 10

Spleen 9

Spleen 6

Stomach 41

Liver 3

Bladder 40

Bladder 57

FIGURE 12
Leg points.

There are many points and nerves used in the study of dim-mak. Theoretically, any nerve or acupuncture point can be used for an attack. However, not all of the points are accessible and not all nerves will have a major effect when attacked. Only the most commonly used dim-mak points are discussed in this book. (See Figure 13.) For a quick reference guide to the points and their neurological connections, refer to Table 2, which shows the major nerve, spinal segment, and organ affected when each point is attacked. An anatomy atlas and a reliable chart or book on acupuncture are recommended for referencing the points mentioned in this book.

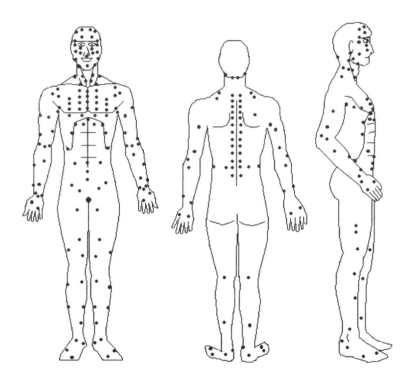

FIGURE 13
Point chart.

Some of the points deserve special mention. The arm points are the most vulnerable and might even be the most important (see fig. 11). The points on the radial nerve are referred to as the lung, triple warmer, and large intestine points. In dim-mak, these are known to affect the lungs. How can points on the radial nerve affect the lungs? The answer lies in the neurological connections of the radial nerve with the lungs and diaphragm. The phrenic nerve controls the diaphragm, which is a muscle located below the lungs that controls a person's ability to breathe. Stimulation of this nerve can cause a spasm of the diaphragm, which can lead to difficulty breathing. Because the radial nerve is connected to the phrenic nerve at the C5 level of the spinal cord, stimulating the radial nerve can cause stimulation of the phrenic nerve, leading to a spasm of the diaphragm and thus difficulty breathing. There is a second neurologic connection that enables the radial nerve to affect the lungs. The radial nerve is connected to the heart and lungs by convergence with the sympathetic nerves at the T1 level of the spinal cord. Pain coming from the lungs can have profound parasympathetic effects on the heart, which can result in a vasovagal faint. The lung sympathetic nerves sense pain in the airways of the lungs. Thus, because the radial nerve is connected to the lung sympathetic nerves through convergence, striking the radial nerve can stimulate the lung sympathetic nerves and cause a vasovagal faint. (See Figure 14.)

The large intestine points along the outer portion of the arm are also on the radial nerve and affect the lungs through the same mechanism. One might question how this nerve affects the large intestine. The answer is simple and lies in the radial nerve's connection with the phrenic nerve. As stated, the phrenic nerve can cause the diaphragm to go into a spasm. If the diaphragm, which rests on top of the transverse portion of the large intestine, is in a spasm, it can irritate the large intestine, disrupting its normal function. When the large intestine is irritated, the body increases the movement of waste through it as a means of eliminating the irritant. This

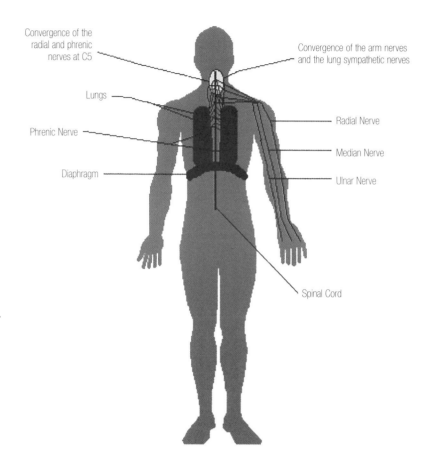

Convergence of the radial and phrenic nerves at C5

Convergence of the arm nerves and the lung sympathetic nerves

Lungs

Phrenic Nerve

Diaphragm

Radial Nerve

Median Nerve

Ulnar Nerve

Spinal Cord

FIGURE 14
The convergence of the arm nerves with the lung sympathetic nerves and phrenic nerve.

explains why the large intestine points can cause an increase in bowel motility.

The median nerve is located in the middle of the inner arm and is attacked through the pericardial points. This nerve has a direct connection to the heart through its convergence with the cardiac sympathetic nerves. Pericardium 6 is one of the easiest points to attack and is used extensively in dim-mak, normally in combination with other points that affect the heart. The ulnar nerve is also located on the medial aspect of the forearm and connects to the spine at C7, C8, and T1. This nerve is attacked through the heart points on the arm and is also connected to the sympathetic nerves of the heart at T1. (See Figures 11 and 15.) Because of their connection with the cardiac sympathetic nerves, the heart and pericardial points located on the ulnar and median nerves can adversely affect the heart when attacked.

The points that affect the heart are the most effective, but they are also the most dangerous. (The subject of attacking the heart will be covered in detail in a later section.) Attacking points on the ulnar and median nerves can also cause a somatovisceral reflex and increased sympathetic nervous system activity. Both of these effects can cause a spasm of the coronary arteries. When a spasm of the coronary arteries is severe or occurs in the area of an arthrosclerotic plaque, it can cause a drastic reduction in blood flow to the heart, resulting in a heart attack. Normally, such a severe constriction of the coronary arteries can only be caused by very strong stimulation of the cardiac sympathetic nerves. This means that usually one would have to attack multiple points with synergistic effects on the heart to cause a heart attack. However, a heart attack is always a possibility when attacking the heart points, especially if the recipient of the attack has preexisting heart disease. A less extreme effect of attacks to points on the ulnar and median nerves can be knockout resulting from simulated cardiac pain.

Some of the points on the chest and back can affect more than one organ. (See Figure 10.) This is due to the convergence of sympathetic nerves from more than one internal organ connecting to the same level of the spinal cord. When a point is attacked, a neurological signal is transmitted to a specific level of the spinal cord. If that level is connected to

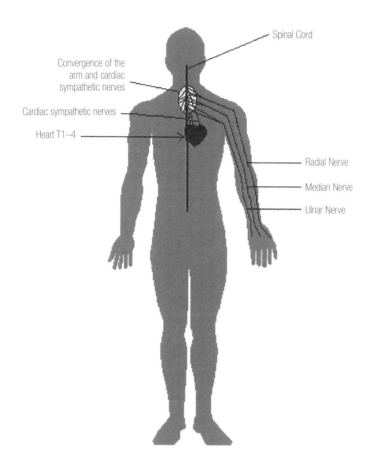

Spinal Cord

Convergence of the
arm and cardiac
sympathetic nerves

Cardiac sympathetic nerves

Heart T1–4

Radial Nerve

Median Nerve

Ulnar Nerve

FIGURE 15
The convergence of the arm nerves and the cardiac sympathetic nerves.

more than one internal organ, the point could affect any of the connecting organs. Such points will be referred to as combination points. All of the points on the first four intercostal nerves, the first four dorsal nerve roots, and the celiac plexus are included in this group. All of the points on these nerves are located on the chest and back and include Lung 1–2,

Stomach 15–17, Conception Vessel 14, 17–20, Gall Bladder 22–23, Spleen 17, Kidney 23–26, Bladder 11–14, and Pericardium 4.

The combination points can be set up to affect different organs because of the neurological phenomena of convergence and facilitation. For instance, attacking the ulnar or median nerves will facilitate the cardiac sympathetic nerves, which will cause the combination points connected to T1–4 to affect the heart. Likewise, attacking the radial nerve will facilitate the lung sympathetic nerves and thereby cause the same points to affect the lung.

Aberrant reference combinations can be thought of as being similar to combination points in this regard. If an aberrant reference combination affects a spinal level connected to the sympathetic nerves of more than one internal organ, it will affect the organs whose sympathetic nerves were facilitated. For example, an aberrant reference combination that facilitated the T4 level of the spinal cord would affect the heart if the cardiac sympathetic nerves were facilitated either before or during the attack. However, if the lung sympathetic nerves were facilitated before or during the attack, the same combination would affect the lungs instead.

Conception Vessel 14 is a particularly powerful combination point that can affect many of the internal organs, including the heart. The location of this point correlates with the location of the celiac plexus, which is a relay station for the sympathetic nerves connected to the stomach, intestines, gall bladder, liver, and spleen. Striking this point can produce a pain signal that could seem to be coming from any one of these organs. When a prior dim-mak point or combination facilitates the sympathetic nerves of an internal organ, a strike to the celiac plexus will affect that organ. When this point is attacked without any other points, it can cause diffuse pain in the abdominal organs. This can cause an increase in the activity to the parasympathetic nervous system, leading to a drop in blood pressure and a knockout (vasovagal faint).

Because of these effects, it can be used synergistically before or after any other point that stimulates the parasympathetic nervous system. In addition, when this point is attacked, the intercostal muscles, the diaphragm, and the abdominal muscles all contract to protect the internal organs. This is an unconscious reflex that can cause the subject to have difficulty breathing. The Conception Vessel 14 point can affect the heart because it is connected to the T5 level of the spinal cord, which is directly connected to the cardiac sympathetic nerves. Attacking the celiac plexus can also affect the heart indirectly because of its effects on the parasympathetic nervous system. Because of its multiple effects, the celiac plexus can be used as a vasovagal faint point, a follow-up point, a combination point, and a heart point.

In this book, the heart points have been grouped according to their effects on the heart (see fig. 16). The points that increase the parasympathetic effects on the heart are called the parasympathetic heart points (see fig. 17). The points that increase the sympathetic effects on the heart are called the sympathetic heart points (see fig. 18). Finally, the points that can be used to attack the heart directly through the chest wall are called the autonomic heart points (see fig. 19). Note that the autonomic heart points have different effects depending on whether they are set up by the sympathetic or parasympathetic nervous systems.

All of the points on the front and sides of the body are located on the intercostal nerves or their branches (see fig. 10). Located just under each of the ribs, the intercostal nerves enter the spinal cord at a level that corresponds to their rib number. Like attacks to points located on the arm nerves, attacks to the points on the intercostal nerves can cause pain that affects an internal organ because they are connected to the internal organs by convergence. This means that they can cause a vasovagal faint and a somatovisceral reflex.

Some of the points are located on nerves that can be used for revival. The actual methods of reversing the effects of dim-

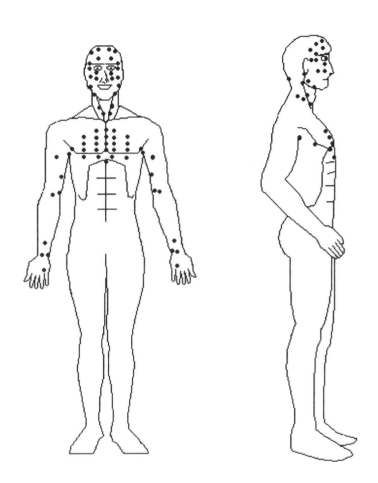

FIGURE 16
Heart points.

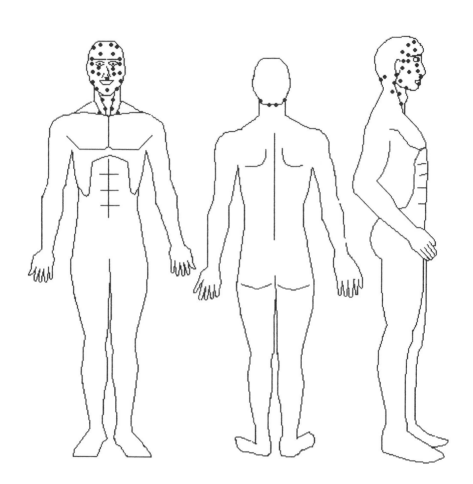

FIGURE 17
Parasympathetic heart points.

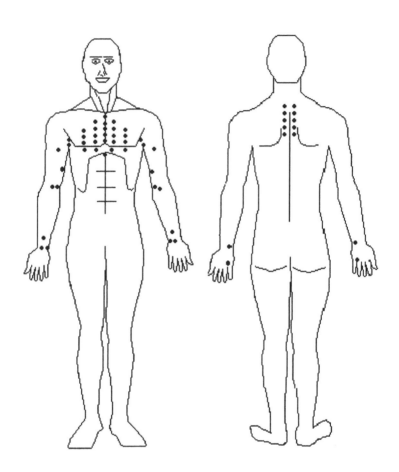

FIGURE 18
Sympathetic heart points.

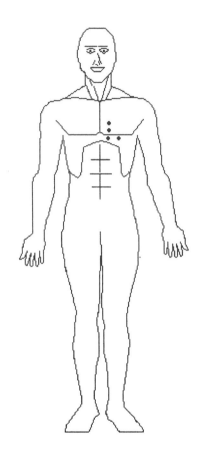

FIGURE 19
Autonomic heart points.

mak will be discussed in the section on revival, but the bladder points deserve special mention here. The bladder points are extremely important and are useful for healing as well as harming (see Table 2 and fig. 4). They are located directly over the dorsal nerve roots, which are connected to the sympathetic nerves from the internal organs. A hard strike to the bladder points will cause a direct increase in the sympathetic stimulation of the corresponding internal organ. On the other hand, firm, steady pressure on these points will decrease the sympathetic stimulation of the corresponding organ and can be used to reverse some of dim-mak's effects. The bladder points are sometimes struck lightly during revival to purposely increase the sympathetic stimulation of an organ.

Not all of the points will affect the internal organs through the nervous system. Some of the dim-mak points can cause direct trauma to the internal organs because they are located directly over the organs. These points, which will be referred to as the organ trauma points, can be used for either a direct attack to the internal organs or a delayed death strike. The organ trauma points include Spleen 13, struck bilaterally to attack the ovaries; Spleen 16 and Liver 13, struck on the right to attack the Liver; Stomach 25, struck bilaterally to attack the intestines; Stomach 20 and 21, struck on the left to attack the stomach; Conception Vessel 6 to attack the bladder; and Bladder 23 and 51 to attack the kidneys.

TABLE 2:
THE NEUROLOGICAL
EFFECTS OF DIM-MAK POINTS

Acupuncture Name	Major Nerve Name	Spinal Level	Organ Affected
Head			
Gall Bladder 13–18	Trigeminal	Cranial Nerve	Brain
Gall Bladder 1–5	Facial	Cranial Nerve	Brain
Small Intestine 18	Trigeminal & Facial	Cranial Nerve	Brain
Small Intestine 17	Facial & Superior Cervical Ganglion	Cranial Nerve	Brain
Triple Warmer 17, 23	Facial	Cranial Nerve	Brain
Stomach 5, 6, 7	Facial	Cranial Nerve	Brain
Conception Vessel 24	Facial	Cranial Nerve	Brain
Governing Vessel 24, 26	Trigeminal	Cranial Nerve	Brain
Gall Bladder 2	Facial	Cranial Nerve	Brain
Gall Bladder 20	Greater Occipital	C3	Diaphragm, Brain
Bladder 10	Lesser Occipital	C3	Diaphragm, Brain
Large Intestine 18	Lessor Occipital/Accessory	C3	Diaphragm, Brain
Neck			
Stomach 9	Carotid Sinus	Cranial Nerve	Heart & Baroreceptor
Small Intestine 16	Great Auricular	C3	Diaphragm
Stomach 10	Cardiac Branch of Vagus	C3	Heart
Large Intestine 17	Stellate Ganglion & Phrenic	C4	Diaphragm
Stomach 11, 12	Supraclavicular	C4	Diaphragm
Torso			
Lung 1	1st Intercostal	T1	Heart, Lung
Conception Vessel 20	1st Intercostal	T1	Heart, Lung
Kidney 26	1st Intercostal	T1	Heart, Lung
Stomach 15	2nd Intercostal	T2	Heart, Lung
Conception Vessel 19	2nd Intercostal	T2	Heart, Lung
Kidney 25	2nd Intercostal	T2	Heart, Lung
Stomach 16	3rd Intercostal	T3	Heart, Lung
Conception Vessel 18	3rd Intercostal	T3	Heart, Lung

Kidney 24	3rd Intercostal	T3	Heart, Lung
Stomach 17	4th Intercostal	T4	Heart, Lung
Gall Bladder 22	4th Intercostal	T4	Heart, Lung
Pericardium 1	4th Intercostal	T4	Heart, Lung
Conception Vessel 17	4th Intercostal	T4	Heart, Lung
Kidney 23	4th Intercostal	T4	Heart, Lung
Gall Bladder 23	5th Intercostal	T5	Heart, Lung
Stomach 18	5th Intercostal	T5	Heart, Lung, Liver (R)
Spleen 17	5th Intercostal	T5	Heart, Lung
Kidney 22	5th Intercostal	T5	Heart, Lung
Conception Vessel 14	5th Intercostal/Celiac plexus	T5–9	Heart, Stomach, Intestines
Liver 14	6th Intercostal	6	Stomach, Gall Bladder (R)
Spleen 21	7th Intercostal	T7	Stomach, Intestines, Spleen (L)
Gall Bladder 24	7th Intercostal	T7	Stomach, Intestines, Spleen (L)
Liver 13	10th Intercostal	T10	Large Intestine, Genitourinary
Gall Bladder 25	11th Intercostal	T11	Large Intestine, Genitourinary
Conception Vessel 6	11th Intercostal	T11	Large Intestine, Genitourinary
Liver 12	Ilioinguinal	L1	Large Intestine, Genitourinary
Spleen 12	Femoral	L1	Large Intestine, Genitourinary

Back

Triple Warmer 15	Accessory, Suprascapular	C5	Heart, Lung, Cranial Nerve
Gall Bladder 21	Accessory, Suprascapular	C5	Heart, Lung, Cranial Nerve
Small Intestine 11	Suprascapular, 5th Dorsal Root	C5/T5	Heart, Lung
Bladder 11	1st Dorsal Nerve Root	T1	Heart, Lung, Head/Neck, Trachea
Bladder 12	2nd Dorsal Nerve Root	T2	Heart, Lung, Head/Neck, Trachea
Bladder 13	3rd Dorsal Nerve Root	T3	Heart, Lung, Head/Neck, Trachea
Bladder 14	4th Dorsal Nerve Root	T4	Heart, Lung, Head/Neck Trachea
Bladder 15	5th Dorsal Nerve Root	T5	Heart, Lung, Liver (R), Aorta
Bladder 16	6th Dorsal Nerve Root	T6	Stomach, Gall Bladder (R)
Bladder 17	7th Dorsal Nerve Root	T7	Stomach, Spleen (L) Pancreas (R)
Bladder 18	8th Dorsal Nerve Root	T8	Stomach, Small Intestine
Bladder 19	9th Dorsal Nerve Root	T9	Stomach, Small Intestine
Bladder 20	10th Dorsal Nerve Root	T10	Small Intestine Kidney, Gonads
Bladder 21	11th Dorsal Nerve Root	T11	Small Intestine Kidney, Gonads
Bladder 22	12th Dorsal Nerve Root	T12	Appendix, Colon, Bladder, Prostate
Bladder 23	1st Lumbar Root	L1	Colon, Kidney, Bladder, Genitals

Arm

Lung 5, 6, 7, 8	Radial	C5	Heart, Lung
Pericardium 2	Musculocutaneous	C5	Heart, Lung
Large Intestine 10, 11	Radial	C6	Heart, Lung
Large Intestine 12, 13, 14	Radial	C6	Heart, Lung
Large Intestine 4, 5, 6	Radial	C6	Heart, Lung
Triple Warmer 11, 12	Radial	C6	Heart, Lung
Pericardium 3, 6, 7	Median	T1	Heart, Lung
Heart 1,2,3, 6	Ulnar	T1	Heart, Lung
Small Intestine 6	Ulnar	T1	Heart, Lung

Leg

Spleen 11	Femoral	L2	Colon, Bladder, Genitals
Liver 11	Femoral	L2	Femoral Vein
Gall Bladder 31	Femoral	L3	None Directly
Spleen 10	Femoral	L3	None Directly
Stomach 34	Femoral	L4	None Directly
Spleen 6	Tibial	L4	Great Saphenous Vein
Spleen 9	Tibial	L4	Great Saphenous Vein
Liver 6	Femoral	L4	Great Saphenous Vein
Kidney 6	Femoral/Saphenous	L4	Great Saphenous Vein
Kidney 8	Femoral/Saphenous	L4	Great Saphenous Vein
Stomach 38	Femoral/Saphenous	L5	Great Saphenous Vein
Gall Bladder 41	Peroneal	L5	None Directly
Liver 3	Peroneal	L5	None Directly
Stomach 41	Peroneal	L5	None Directly
Stomach 36	Peroneal	L5	None Directly
Bladder 57, 60, 62	Tibial/Sural	S1	Lesser Saphenous Vein
Bladder 40	Tibial	S1	Popliteal Vein
Gall Bladder 39	Peroneal	S1	None Directly

Organ

Ovaries
Liver
Intestines
Stomach
Bladder
Kidney

Trauma Points

Spleen 13 Bilaterally
Spleen 16 and Liver 13 on Right
Stomach 25 bilaterally
Stomach 20 and 21 on Left
Conception Vessel 4, 5, 6
Bladder 23 and 52 Bilaterally

MULTIPLE POINTS

The number of points to strike is questionable. It has already been mentioned that multiple points can have synergistic effects based on the phenomena of summation and facilitation. It follows logically that adding more points to a combination increases the probability of severe damage. In some cases, striking with the correct angle and force can cause a vasovagal faint with just one point. However, it is much easier to cause a knockout using multiple points. Inducing a stimulus strong enough to cause cardiac arrest or a severe somatovisceral reflex resulting in a heart attack or organ failure usually requires the use of multiple points. Although the exact number used by the ancient masters remains a mystery, there is a scientific basis for using combinations of two, three, and five points.

When two nerves are stimulated at the same time, the phenomenon of aberrant reference causes the body to interpret the pain as coming from somewhere in the middle. Thus, if one were to strike two points located on the body, the pain would register in the middle. If this midway point corresponded to the location of an internal organ, a vasovagal faint and possibly a somatovisceral reflex could result. An example would be striking Liver 13 on both sides simultaneously. The body interprets such a stimulus as coming from the large intestine because the Liver 13 point is on the 10th intercostal nerve, which connects to the spinal cord at T10. The large intestine sympathetic nerves connect to this same level. Thus, the pain from the Liver 13 points will cause severe pain in the large intestine, leading to a vasovagal faint. Combining any two points that can cause pain in the heart, lung, digestive tract, bladder, or genitals due to aberrant reference can result in this type of knockout.

What happens when three or more points are attacked? At the most basic level, this could also cause a knockout. Medical science has found that a vasovagal faint can be caused by excessive neural traffic in an area of the brain called the nucleus tractus solitarii.[1] This area receives neurological stimulation from many sources. Nerve pain can stimulate this area indirectly, and some of the points are located on nerves that can stimulate this area directly. Striking points on three or more nerves simultaneously sends a barrage of pain signals to the nucleus tractus solitarii, causing excessive neural traffic, which results in a vasovagal faint. This will not occur with just any three nerves; the nerves must have synergistic effects or cause severe pain.

At a more advanced level, combinations of three or more points affecting the heart could cause death due to cardiac arrest, a heart attack, or an irregular heartbeat. In addition to causing organ failure, attacks to three or more points that affect the other internal organs can cause cardiac arrest as well as organ failure. Severe pain in the internal organs can cause a drastic increase in the parasympathetic effects on the heart, which usually leads to a vasovagal faint but can also result in cardiac arrest.

Some have suggested that attacking five or more points can cause death. Based on the five elements relating to the meridians of acupuncture, it has been postulated that attacking five points following the cycle of destruction can cause death. At this time, there is no scientific evidence to support this. However, there are five basic methods of combining points in a synergistic manner that are based on medical science. Thus, in order to be able to cause maximum damage based on the concepts of medical science, one must attack at least five points.

Set-up Points

The teaching of dim-mak has always stressed the use of set-up points, which was believed to work by affecting a person's energy flow. The application of medical science to the study of dim-mak can provide a modern scientific explanation for the efficacy of the set-up points. There are several different methods of setting up the dim-mak points, and there is a slightly different explanation for each. The methods range from a simple nerve attack causing pain to very specific nerve combinations affecting a certain level of the spinal cord. The advanced methods are based on aberrant reference, facilitation, and summation (refer to Chapter 2 for a review of these concepts).

The different methods will be discussed in detail, but try not to get bogged down with the specifics of each nerve and point, since some of this has already been discussed. It is the interrelationships of the nerves and how the concepts of medical science apply to them that are important. An understanding of these aspects will enable one to set up any dim-mak point.

The simplest method of setting up an attack involves attacking points on the arm or leg nerves to activate the sympathetic nervous system (see figs. 11 and 12). The use of pain to set up certain nerves is based on a reflex called a somatosympathetic reflex. Actually, pain from any nerve can cause this effect, but the arm and leg nerves are particularly vulnerable. Medical research has shown that an increase in the activity of the sympathetic nervous system magnifies the effects of the parasympathetic nervous system on the heart.[2] Thus, this method potentiates any point that affects the parasympathetic nervous system (see figs. 9 and 17). (The points that affect the parasympathetic system will be discussed in a later section.)

A more advanced method involves setting up a specific organ or spinal level. This is accomplished by applying the concepts of facilitation and convergence. Since the arms are usually vulnerable when an opponent reaches to grab or strike, the heart points on the ulnar and median nerves will be discussed first. Attacking the ulnar and median nerves through the heart and pericardial points will adversely affect the heart as well as set up the other heart points. It will also set up the combination points to affect the heart. When the ulnar and median nerves are stimulated, all the nerves that enter the spinal cord at T1–5 will become facilitated. This includes the cardiac sympathetic nerves, which will cause the celiac plexus, the first five intercostal nerves, and the first five dorsal nerve roots to have a greater effect on the heart when attacked. The effects of attacking points on these nerves can include a vasovagal faint, cardiac arrest, and a heart attack. As additional heart points are added, the probability of seriously injuring the heart increases dramatically.

The same principles apply to the lung, large intestine, and triple warmer points on the radial nerve. When this nerve is attacked, the nerves that connect to the spinal cord at C5–T4 become facilitated. This includes the phrenic nerve, the first four dorsal nerve roots, and the first four intercostal nerves. Stimulation of the radial nerve will cause the points on these nerves to affect the lung instead of the heart. This occurs because the lung sympathetic nerves are facilitated by an attack to the radial nerve. The effects of attacking points on these nerves can include a vasovagal faint or cardiac arrest.

The phenomenon of aberrant reference can be exploited to set up certain points. When two nerves are stimulated simultaneously, the spinal cord will become facilitated in the middle of where the two nerves connect to the spinal cord. Thus, an aberrant reference combination will set up points that are connected to the facilitated segment of the spinal cord. For example, if one were to stimulate a heart point on the ulnar nerve in combination with the Liver 12 point on the ilioinguinal nerve, the pain would register at the T6–7 level of the spine. This would set up the stomach, the 6th intercostal nerve at Liver 14, the celiac plexus at Conception Vessel 14, and the 6th dorsal nerve root at Bladder 16. Because the effects of these points are potentiated, attacking these points could result in cardiac arrest at the worst and a vasovagal faint at the least. In addition, because the parasympathetic effects are increased, any point that can increase the parasympathetic effects on the heart will be potentiated because of summation.

The phenomenon of summation offers another method of setting up the points. One could attack multiple nerves with synergistic effects if they all connected to the spinal cord at the same level or affected the same part of the central nervous system. An example would be an attack that uses aberrant reference (combination of arm and leg points) to cause facilitation at T6. The follow-up could include a simultaneous attack to any of the nerves connected to T6 (including the same points mentioned in the previous example). This example illustrates the use of summation to potentiate an attack that was set up by the use of aberrant reference.

In summary, there are multiple methods of setting up the dim-mak points, all of which can be explained by medical science. The simplest method involves nerve pain caused by a single point. This sets up the parasympathetic mediated points because of somatosympathetic reflexes. The second method involves attacking the nerves of the arm to set up the heart and lungs. The points on the ulnar and median nerves will set up the points on the first five intercostal nerves and the first five dorsal nerve roots to affect the heart. The points on the radial nerve will set up the first four intercostal nerves and the first four dorsal nerve roots to affect the lung. The third method involves attacking a particular spinal segment to cause facilitation. This increases the vulnerability of the nerves that are connected to the facilitated level. One can use an aberrant reference technique or a direct attack to the nerves connected to a specific level of the spinal cord. Finally, summation can be used to set up the points. At an advanced level, one could combine these methods of setting up the points to achieve an even greater effect.

Chapter 4

Methods of Attacking

T here are many different methods of attacking the dim-mak points. The specific methods of striking and grabbing the points are beyond the scope of this book. However, this section will discuss a few general concepts that apply to all methods of attacking the points. These include the vulnerability of the nervous system, the angle and direction of an attack, and the actual attacking of the nerves. The best method of learning dim-mak is through the practice and study of the traditional forms. The concepts mentioned here will guide the martial artist in finding the dim-mak applications contained within the traditional forms.

One must consider the vulnerability of the nervous system when analyzing methods of attacking the points. The exposed portions of a nerve are usually located in a body cavity between muscles, bones, or both. One can usually find a sore spot in the location of the point. Although it is possible to learn the location of the points from books and charts, following the guidance of an authentic teacher and learning the point locations from experience are advisable. The practice of massage, or shiatsu, is another very useful tool for learning the locations of the points, as it enables one to quickly learn the location and depth of the points without causing any harm.

The second area of concern is the angle and direction of the dim-mak attacks. Usually a person will strike into the cavity, or towards the center of the body. However, in order to get maximum stimulation of a nerve, the attacking method should either stretch the nerve or compress it against a bone. The most effective methods of attack involve both. If a nerve is located in close proximity to a bone, the attack should strike or grind the nerve into the bone. If a nerve is located in an area that is soft, then the attack should be penetrating to stretch the nerve. It is also important to consider the area of the body that is being attacked. If striking a soft area, one should use a very pointed surface, such as the fingertips, toes, or a single knuckle. If striking a hard area, one should use a striking surface that has more tissue to protect it, such as the palm or the edge of the hand.

These first two concepts offer guidelines for developing effective dim-mak attacks. However, they require a basic understanding of anatomy. An easier method involves analyzing the traditional forms (kata) for hidden dim-mak applications because they usually contain the correct order, angle, and direction of attacking the points. Once it is determined how the points can be attacked with a specific technique, it is easy to figure out which points would work best. They are usually those that enable one to compress and stretch the nerves in a synergistic manner. The caveat is that one must first learn the correct execution of the traditional forms from an authentic teacher. Performing the techniques of a form incorrectly can make it quite difficult to find the correct dim-mak applications.

There are other benefits to be gained from kata practice. When executed correctly, forms help a student develop body control and the ability to focus all of one's energy into a technique. Some call the latter skill focus, and others describe it as the harnessing of internal power. Whatever the description, this is an essential component of dim-mak. Focus is usually achieved by imagining the correct dim-mak applications while practicing forms. Because the subconscious mind does not differentiate between a mental picture and an actual event, visualizing an attack enables one to train the mind as if he or she were actually being attacked. Such training prepares one to respond to a real threat by attacking the points without any conscious thought.

The last concept to be addressed is the actual striking of the nerves. The points must be struck very hard for full effect. The effect created with a nerve strike should be similar to that of striking one's finger with a hammer. When a painful stimulus is applied to a nerve, the brain can perceive it as a superficial pain, a deep pain, or both. The peripheral nerves are actually multiple nerve fibers grouped together. Within this bundle, there are two types of nerve fibers that transmit pain: type A and type C. Type A nerves are responsible for a fast, sharp pain that is localized to a specific area. These fibers have a low threshold and can be activated with a minimal stimulus. They send impulses to the brain in what is called the neospinalthalamic tract of the spinal cord. In this pathway, there are no connections to the medulla or hypothalamus, which are the areas of the brain that are responsible for controlling the autonomic nervous system. Thus, pain in the type A nerve fibers has no effect on the autonomic nervous system.

The type C nerves are responsible for a severe, deep pain that is associated with autonomic effects such as nausea, perspiration, and blood pressure changes. These autonomic changes are explained by the neurological connections between type C nerves and the brain. Pain from the type C nerves is transmitted to the brain in the paleospinalthalamic tract of the spinal cord. This tract has direct connections to the medulla and hypothalamus. Since the effects of dim-mak occur through the autonomic nervous system, the type C nerves must be stimulated when a point is attacked. These nerves have a high threshold and only respond to a very strong stimulus.

In order to activate as many type C nerve fibers as possible, one should strike the points with a snapping action. This magnifies the perceived power of the attack. As stated, each peripheral nerve is composed of multiple nerve fibers. Within each bundle of nerve fibers, there are multiple type C nerves with different thresholds. Some of these nerves will discharge with a fairly moderate strike and others require much more force. If one were to slowly press on a point with increasing amounts of force, eventually many of the high threshold C nerves would be stimulated. However, by the time the higher threshold nerves were stimulated, many of the lower threshold nerves would be in a refractory state. This means that they would be unable to fire until they reset their electric charge (ionic polarity). When a point is struck with a quick snapping strike, many of the high and low threshold type C nerves fire at the same time. The increased number of nerve fibers transmitting signals magnifies the pain of the attack, which results in a much greater effect on the autonomic nervous system.

Another method of maximally stimulating the type C nerves involves attacking the same point many times. This too can lead to greater pain and increased autonomic effects. The potentiation of a nerve attack by repeated stimulation occurs at three different areas of the nervous system: the nerve, the synapse, and the spinal cord. The potentiation at the level of the nerve occurs by two mechanisms. The first is damage to the nerve, which causes it to become hyper-responsive to pain.[1] The second involves the recruitment of additional nerve fibers to increase the number of signals sent to the spinal cord. The human nervous system monitors the intensity of a painful stimulus by the number of neurons that send signals to the brain in combination with the frequency of the signals. A very painful stimulus activates a large number of nerve fibers. Repeated stimulation of a nerve increases the number of nerve fibers that send signals to the spinal cord.

Thus, repeated stimulation of a nerve will cause increased pain because more nerve fibers will be activated and the nerve itself will become hyperresponsive.

The synapse is the second area where a nerve attack can be potentiated by repeated stimulation. Nerves communicate with each other by chemicals. When a nerve is stimulated, it releases chemicals that travel across the synapse and stimulate the adjacent nerve. Repeated stimulation of a nerve results in a 60-second interval of enhanced pain in the adjacent nerve because it becomes hyperresponsive. This occurs because there is a buildup of calcium in the adjacent nerve. This is called post-tetanic potentiation and means that the effect of a nerve strike will be potentiated when one strikes the same nerve within 60 seconds of the first strike.

The third area where repeated attacks to a nerve can cause potentiation is in the spinal cord. Pain enters the spinal cord in an area called the dorsal horn. Repetitive stimulation of the type C nerves causes the nerve cells in the spinal cord to increase their rate of discharge until a state of constant nerve activity is reached.[2] At this point, even the slightest stimulation of a type C nerve will cause excruciating pain because the spinal cord is hyperactive. In other words, the spinal segment becomes facilitated.

In summary, when one strikes the same nerve numerous times, the effect is magnified for the following four reasons:

- The number of nerve fibers transmitting the pain signal is increased.
- The injured nerve up-regulates its sodium channels and becomes hyperresponsive.
- The adjacent nerve becomes hyperresponsive due to post-tetanic potentiation.
- The spinal cord pain pathway becomes hyperresponsive due to facilitation.

Since these effects usually occur in graduated steps, one

must strike a nerve at least three times to magnify the effects at all levels. To put all of this very simply, if one strikes a nerve and the effect is minimal, one could restrike the same nerve multiple times to potentiate the effect. This potentiation of a dim-mak point with repetitive stimulation is often exploited at seminars. In cases where an individual is able to cause drastic effects after lightly tapping a point, usually the point was touched, pressed, and tapped multiple times prior to the "light tap."

There are many different methods of attacking the dim-mak points. These are just general guidelines to enable one to find the dim-mak applications hidden within the traditional forms. Again, the beginner is advised to follow the instruction of an experienced teacher. There are certain basic components of the martial arts that one needs to learn before attempting to study the relationship between dim-mak and the traditional forms. At the advanced level, the martial artist should learn the principles behind the techniques in order to develop his or her own methods. It was this approach that led to the creation of dim-mak in the first place. At a very advanced level, two different masters might attack the same point with slightly different methods. In fact, the variations in the katas of different styles are the result of different masters refining their techniques.

Chapter 5

A Medical Knockout

Perhaps the most intriguing aspect of dim-mak is the pressure point knockout. Those who have witnessed such a feat are usually amazed at how easily a person is knocked unconscious as well as how little force is used. This form of knockout is unique to dim-mak and is quite different from the classic boxing knockout, where one is struck in the head causing a concussion. The pressure point knockout has more in common with fainting than boxing. In fact, when a person faints at the sight of blood or upon hearing bad news, the body undergoes almost the same changes in blood pressure and heart rate as it does during a pressure point knockout. The mechanism of the pressure point knockout involves changes in the autonomic nervous system that cause a sudden drop in blood pressure leading to a loss of consciousness.

Vasovagal faint (syncope) is the medical term for a loss of consciousness due to a sudden drop in blood pressure. A vasovagal reaction is defined as a drop in blood pressure with lightheadedness, nausea, and vomiting but no loss of consciousness. It has been found that during a vasovagal faint there is a sudden dilation of the blood vessels in combination with a decrease in heart rate. This causes an acute drop in blood pressure leading to decreased blood perfusion of the brain. In response to this, the blood vessels in the brain constrict, leading to a further decrease in blood perfusion.[1] This dramatic decrease in blood perfusion causes the brain to be deprived of oxygen and leads to a loss of consciousness.

The manner in which the autonomic nervous system induces a sudden drop in blood pressure is quite complex. Normally there is a partial constriction of the peripheral blood vessels due to a constant signal from the sympathetic nervous system. When the body needs to increase blood pressure, it increases the stimulation of the sympathetic nervous system. This causes the heart rate to increase and the blood vessels to constrict, leading to an increase in blood pressure. During a vasovagal faint, the parasympathetic nervous system slows or stops the heart and interrupts the sympathetic signal to the major blood vessels, causing them to open wider. The combined effect of the dilated blood vessels and the decreased heart rate is a drastic reduction in blood pressure.

The reason there is a drop in blood pressure when the blood vessels dilate is because there is a larger tube for the blood to flow through. One can think of the comparison between water flowing out of a squeeze bottle with the squirt top on and then suddenly without any top. The pressure coming out would decrease unless one squeezed the bottle harder. In the body, when the blood vessels dilate, the heart normally pumps faster and harder to keep the blood pressure up. During a vasovagal faint, the blood vessels dilate, but the heart rate slows down, which causes the blood pressure to drop.

There are many different methods of inducing a vasovagal faint. The exact mechanism of how this occurs is complicated, but the basic neurologic connections will be outlined here. Try not to become overwhelmed with the neuroscience involved; the important concept is that there are neurological connections between the dim-mak points and the area of the brain that can cause a vasovagal faint.

All of the dim-mak methods that cause a knockout stimulate an area of the brain called the nucleus tractus solitarii. Medical research has found that excessive neural traffic in this area can cause a vasovagal faint.[2] The nucleus tractus solitarii is responsible for the increased activity of the parasympathetic nervous system and the withdrawal of the sympathetic signal to the blood vessels. This occurs through a number of mechanisms. One involves the inhibition of areas in the vasomotor center of the brain. There are two areas called the reticularis gigantocellularis and the reticularis parvicellularis that have been found to cause high blood pressure when stimulated.[3] Normally the nucleus tractus solitarii inhibits these areas and maintains the blood pressure in a normal range.[4] When the nucleus tractus solitarii is stimulated, there is excessive inhibition of these areas, which causes an interruption of the sympathetic signal supplying the blood vessels. The result is an increase in the diameter of the blood vessels and a decrease in blood pressure. At the same time, the nucleus tractus solitarii stimulates the motor nucleus of the vagus nerve, leading to an increase in the parasympathetic effects on the heart. This causes the simultaneous decrease in the heart rate.

The nucleus tractus solitarii can be stimulated in three different ways in order to induce a vasovagal faint. Applying the concept of aberrant reference, it can be stimulated indirectly by using dim-mak point combinations to simulate pain in some of the internal organs. Another option involves causing pain in the type C nerves, which stimulates the nucleus tractus solitarii indirectly through the hypothalamus. The type C nerves can be attacked through most of the dim-mak points, but extreme force is required to do so. Finally, attacking points on the carotid sinus, trigeminal nerve, facial nerve, glossopharnygeal nerve, vagus nerve, optic nerve, and the occipital nerves can stimulate the nucleus tractus solitarii directly. Each of these methods will be discussed separately.

First, the phenomenon of aberrant reference can be used to cause pain in the heart, lungs, digestive tract, bladder, or genitals. For example, if one stimulated two nerves that facilitated the T9 level of the spinal cord, the pain could be perceived as coming from the intestines. If the pain were strong enough, the result would be a vasovagal faint. An aberrant reference combination will have this effect whenever it causes simulated pain in one of the organs mentioned. In addition, because a vasovagal faint is associated with increased parasympathetic effects on the heart, any combination of points that causes a vasovagal faint will also cause an increase in the parasympathetic effects on the heart.

The concept of convergence can be used to achieve the same effect. Very strong stimulation of a peripheral nerve can cause the brain to think the pain is coming from the internal organ that the nerve was connected to by convergence. If the pain is in one of the organs mentioned, the result could be a vasovagal faint. For example, if one stimulated the ulnar nerve, the brain might perceive the pain as coming from the heart because the ulnar nerve and the heart are both connected to the spinal cord at T1 (see fig. 15). It should be noted that convergence and aberrant reference are synergistic when used together; however, the resultant enhanced parasympathetic effects on the heart could lead to cardiac arrest.

The easiest method of causing a vasovagal faint involves stimulating points on nerves that can directly stimulate the nucleus tractus solitarii. All of these nerves can cause a vasovagal faint as well as a very strong increase in parasympathetic nervous system activity that can lead to very serious parasympathetic mediated effects such as heart block and cardiac arrest. It all depends on how strongly the nerves are stimulated. When such nerves are set up or used in combination, they are much more likely to cause a vasovagal faint or cardiac arrest. The points located on the following nerves can all be attacked to cause a vasovagal faint directly. They include cranial nerves 2, 5, 7, 9, and 10; the greater and lesser occipital nerves; and the carotid sinus. (See Figures 9 and 17.)

CAROTID SINUS

The body closely monitors the blood pressure through various mechanisms. Baroreceptors are sensory organs located in the carotid arteries, the aorta, and the chambers of the heart. When these receptors sense increased blood pressure, they send a signal to the nucleus tractus solitarii in the brain, leading to a decrease in blood pressure. When the baroreceptors are hyperactive or overstimulated, they can cause a vasovagal faint. In fact, there is a syndrome called carotid sinus syncope consisting of multiple vasovagal fainting attacks due to a hypersensitivity of the carotid sinus. The carotid sinus is the only baroreceptor that is directly vulnerable to attack and is a major target for many dim-mak techniques. Because it can cause a knockout with a minimum of effort, this point is used extensively for demonstration purposes during seminars.

The carotid sinus is found at the bifurcation of the common carotid artery, which correlates with the Stomach 9 point (see fig. 9). When this point is attacked, the carotid sinus sends a false signal to the brain that the blood pressure is extremely high. It also directly stimulates the nucleus tractus solitarii, leading to a vasovagal faint, heart block, or cardiac arrest.

CRANIAL NERVES

The second, fifth, seventh, and tenth cranial nerves are a direct link to the parasympathetic nervous system and are used extensively in dim-mak. The fifth cranial nerve, called the trigeminal nerve, corresponds to many of the dim-mak points on the face. It has three branches that monitor pain in the face and head. There are reports in medical literature of trigeminal neuralgia causing a vasovagal faint as well as cardiac arrest.[5][6] Neuralgia is the medical term for nerve pain. Thus, by striking points on the trigeminal nerve, the martial artist can cause trigeminal neuralgia (trigeminal nerve pain) leading to a vasovagal faint or cardiac arrest. The points on the trigeminal nerve include Gall Bladder 13–18, Stomach 2–3, Bladder 6–8, and Small Intestine 18 (see fig. 9).

The ninth cranial nerve is the glossopharyngeal nerve. There are reports in the medical literature of glossopharyngeal neuralgia causing a vasovagal faint, arrhythmias (irregular heartbeats), and cardiac arrest.[7] This nerve is connected to the carotid sinus, the vagus nerve, the facial nerve, and the superior and middle cervical sympathetic ganglions. Thus, stimulation of points on any of these nerves can also cause a vasovagal faint or cardiac arrest. The superior cervical ganglion is accessible through Small Intestine 17, and the middle cervical ganglion is located under Small Intestine 16 (see fig. 9).

The seventh cranial nerve, also known as the facial nerve, is attacked through following points: Triple Warmer 17 and 23; Small Intestine 17 and 18; Gall Bladder 1, 2, and 3; and Stomach 5, 6, and 7 (see fig. 9). Stimulation of the facial nerve has been found to directly decrease the heart rate via the vagus nerve.[8] In addition, this nerve is directly connected to the trigeminal and glossopharyngeal nerves. Thus, stimulation of the facial nerve can stimulate the trigeminal, glossopharyngeal, and vagus nerves, resulting in a vasovagal faint or cardiac arrest.

OCULOCARDIAC REFLEX

The optic nerve is known as the second cranial nerve. It runs from the eye directly back to the brain and is responsible for the ability to see. Stimulation of the optic nerve can directly increase the parasympathetic effects on the heart. This is called the oculocardiac reflex and is used by physicians to stop some abnormal heart rhythms. When used in this manner, the physician will apply gentle pressure to the eye with the eyelid closed. The oculocardiac reflex can cause a vasovagal faint when the eyeball is pressed or struck hard. This effect is the result of pressure on the whole eye, not just poking a finger in the eye. This is perhaps one of the easiest cranial nerves to stimulate. Even if the eyelid is closed, strong pressure or a strike can still cause a vasovagal faint or cardiac arrest.

THE GREATER AND LESSER OCCIPITAL NERVES

Two nerves that are easily attacked and can cause a vasovagal faint or complete autonomic failure are the greater and lesser occipital nerves. The greater occipital nerve is located under Bladder 10. The lesser occipital nerve is located under Gall Bladder 20 and Large Intestine 18 (see fig. 9). These two nerves enter the spinal cord at the second and third cervical vertebrae and communicate with the trigeminal, vagus, phrenic, and spinal accessory nerves. There are reports in the medical literature of autonomic failure associated with occipital neuralgia (occipital nerve pain).[9] Autonomic failure can cause orthostatic hypotension, which is an inability to maintain blood pressure when standing and often results in fainting. Consequently, when these nerves are stimulated through dim-mak points, they can can cause a sudden drop in blood pressure and a loss of consciousness.

The Gall Bladder 20 points are also known to be revival points for a dim-mak knockout. The healing effects of these points can be explained by medical science. Since severe pain in the occipital nerves can cause autonomic failure, mild pain should be able to inhibit the autonomic nervous system to a lesser degree. This means that they can be used to reverse the effects of dim-mak attacks, particularly those caused by the parasympathetic nervous system. If the parasympathetic system is overactive, such as during a vasovagal faint, firm pressure on these nerves via the Gall Bladder 20 points will decrease its activity and allow the autonomic nervous system to normalize.

All of the nerves that can directly stimulate the nucleus tractus solitarii to cause a vasovagal faint are connected neurologically. Thus, stimulation of any one of these nerves will facilitate the others. In addition, these nerves are synergistic when attacked together, because they all increase the parasympathetic effects on the heart. To put it simply, martial artists should be forewarned that these points, located on the head, face, and carotid sinus, not only have the ability to cause cardiac arrest but, because they work synergistically, are more likely to do so when used in combination.

An increase in the activity of the sympathetic nervous system will potentiate all methods of causing a vasovagal faint. Evidence of this is found in the treatment of people who suffer from multiple vasovagal fainting attacks. These patients are treated with drugs called beta-blockers, which block the effects of the sympathetic nervous system. It has been found that beta-blockers reduce the number of vasovagal fainting episodes suffered by these patients. Because of this, it is believed that increased activity of the sympathetic nervous system is associated with an increased incidence of vasovagal fainting. In addition, medical research has shown that increased sympathetic activity magnifies the effects of the parasympathetic nervous system on the heart.[10] When applied to dim-mak, this means that the martial artist can set up any of the methods that cause vasovagal faint by first stimulating the sympathetic nervous system.

Because the body responds to pain with an increase in the activity of the sympathetic nervous system due to the somatosympathetic reflex, any dim-mak point that causes pain can be used to set up the vasovagal faint points. Pain can also be used to actually cause a vasovagal faint. The type C nerve fibers that are stimulated by a dim-mak attack have a neurological connection to the hypothalamus, which has a neurological connection to the nucleus tractus solitarii. Thus, severe nerve pain caused by a dim-mak strike can indirectly stimulate the nucleus tractus solitarii through the hypothalamus, resulting in a vasovagal faint. Because this method of causing a vasovagal faint is dependent on the opponent's pain threshold, attacking the type C nerves of a single point can produce this effect in some individuals, whereas in others it requires attacking multiple points. In most people, stimulating three nerves simultaneously will cause pain severe enough to cause a vasovagal faint. This is one of the reasons some of the techniques taught at seminars require the martial artist to strike three or more points.

Because the nucleus tractus solitarii is neurologically connected to the cortex of the brain, which controls higher neurological functions such as reasoning, speaking, and abstract thinking, a person's conscious thoughts and emotions can precipitate a vasovagal faint. This is actually quite common. For example, some people faint at the sight of blood or upon hearing bad news. Because of the neurological connection between the cortex and the nucleus tractus solitarii, a person's thoughts can also inhibit a vasovagal faint, which explains why the element of surprise is necessary for some of the dim-mak knockouts. The input from the cortex can block the dim-mak effects on the nucleus tractus solitarii if a person is expecting to be hit on a point. However, if the martial artist attacks multiple points that have been set up, it is very unlikely that the recipient of the attack would be able to prevent the vasovagal faint.

In summary, attacking the dim-mak points to cause a "pressure point knockout" actually results in a vasovagal faint. Some of the dim-mak points are located on nerves that have a direct neurological connection to the area of the brain responsible for this phenomenon. These nerves, which include the vagus, trigeminal, and facial nerves, as well as the carotid sinus and occipital nerves, can be attacked through the dim-mak points on the face, head, and neck to cause a knockout. A vasovagal faint can also be caused by severe pain in three or more nerves or by pain radiating from one of the internal organs. Using an aberrant reference combination or attacking points that are connected to the organs by convergence can cause pain in the internal organs and thus lead to a vasovagal faint. Increased activity of the sympathetic nervous system will increase the effectiveness of any point or combination that can cause a vasovagal faint. In addition, because a vasovagal faint involves excessive parasympathetic effects on the heart, attacks to such points can have very serious consequences. When combinations of points are used to set up these points or when multiple vasovagal faint techniques are used together, the probability of causing cardiac arrest increases dramatically.

Chapter 6

Attacking the Internal Organs

Although the acupuncture points can have a healing effect on many of the internal organs, paradoxically, the same points can be used to attack the internal organs with effects that range from pain and illness to loss of consciousness and death. Although these effects usually occur very quickly, they can be delayed in certain situations. It is conceivable that the origin of the delayed death touch could be connected to situations where the effects of attacking an internal organ were delayed. Although many of the points can be used to attack the internal organs, there are basically three different methods of causing organ damage: inducing changes in the autonomic nervous system, reducing blood perfusion, and inflicting direct trauma.

To fully grasp the medical explanation of dim-mak's effects on the internal organs, it is essential to have a basic understanding of the nervous system. Although most of this information was explained in the chapter on the nervous system it will be reviewed here for the sake of clarity. All of the internal organs are connected to the sympathetic and parasympathetic nervous systems. The sympathetic nerves of the internal organs monitor pain and supply sympathetic stimulation. These nerves fuse with peripheral nerves that are vulnerable to attack through the dim-mak points (see fig. 3). Medical science has found that stimulation of these peripheral nerves can have adverse effects on the internal organs. These effects are known as somatovisceral reflexes, and there are two methods of causing them: by attacking points that are connected to an internal organ by convergence or by using an aberrant reference combination to facilitate the sympathetic nerves of an internal organ.

Doctors have known for more than 150 years that the internal organs can be adversely affected by stimulating the peripheral nervous system.[1] Scientists originally postulated that neurologically induced damage was the result of an abnormal trophic influence from the nervous system.[2] However, more recent research has shown that stimulation of certain areas of the body can cause decreased blood perfusion of the internal organs.[3] It is quite possible that the neurologically induced damage previously believed to be caused by a trophic influence was caused by an alteration in blood perfusion. Every cell in the body is dependent on a constant blood supply to deliver oxygen and nutrients and remove carbon dioxide and cellular waste. A decrease in blood flow can cause organ dysfunction, and a complete interruption of blood flow can cause organ failure and death. Thus, attacking the dim-mak points can stimulate the peripheral nervous system, and the somatovisceral reflexes that result can effectively decrease the blood perfusion of the internal organs, leading to dysfunction and failure.

In order for an organ to fail, the blood flow must be stopped or decreased for a significant amount of time. Chronic stimulation of a nerve that can cause a somatovisceral reflex can produce a sustained decrease in the blood flow to an internal organ. One method of causing chronic nerve stimulation is to strike a point very hard, causing inflammation in the underlying nerve and tissues. This inflammatory response could result in the nerve's being stimulated for up to a week. If the nerve is neurologically connected to the sympathetic nerves of an internal organ, such prolonged stimulation could cause a chronic somatovisceral reflex. Because the resultant decrease in blood perfusion can cause progressive organ dysfunction, this could have delayed effects, including organ failure. Any nerve that is neurologically connected to the sympathetic nerves of the internal organs can be attacked in this manner, but the dorsal nerve roots under the bladder points are especially effective because inflammation in this area can directly stimulate the sympathetic nerves connected to the internal organs.

The most effective method of decreasing the blood perfusion of an internal organ involves combining the effects of a somatovisceral reflex with those of a vasovagal faint. A somatovisceral reflex will decrease the blood flow to a specific internal organ. When this is combined with the sudden drop in blood pressure caused by a vasovagal faint, the decrease in blood perfusion is magnified. The reason for this is that blood perfusion of the internal organs depends on both blood flow and blood pressure. This drastic decrease in blood perfusion is very similar to shock, which is actually defined as the inability of the body to provide sufficient blood perfusion to the internal organs. The only difference is that in this case the decrease in blood perfusion is limited to one organ. Therefore, one can use what is known about shock to predict how the internal organs will be affected by the combination of a somatovisceral reflex and a vasovagal faint. To illustrate this point, let's look at the effects of decreased blood perfusion of the lungs, liver, kidneys, and digestive system.

The human body is dependent on a constant supply of oxygen for survival. The lungs are the organs responsible for extracting oxygen from the air and eliminating carbon dioxide from the body. Decreased blood perfusion of the lungs can cause an accumulation of fluid in the lungs and a decreased ability to oxygenate the blood.[4] As the lungs accumulate fluid they lose their ability to be stretched during breathing and the fluid acts as a barrier to gas exchange. The combined effects of decreased blood oxygen levels and increased lung stiffness increase the work of breathing. This is a progressive effect that will eventually cause respiratory failure and death unless the patient is put on a mechanical ventilator. There is evidence that the lungs can also be directly damaged by the nervous system. Pulmonary edema (fluid in the lungs) has been associated with abnormalities of the autonomic nervous system.[5] Furthermore, research has shown that this could be due to increased activity of the sympathetic nervous system.[6] This is interesting because the points and combinations that can cause a somatovisceral reflex affecting the lungs also stimulate the sympathetic nerves of the lungs. Attacking the points on the radial nerve, the first four intercostal nerves, and the first four dorsal nerve roots can cause a somatovisceral reflex affecting the lungs. However, the points on the first four intercostal nerves and dorsal nerve roots will only affect the lungs when combined with an attack to the radial nerve because they are combination points. An aberrant reference combination facilitating the T1–4 levels of the spinal cord can also cause a somatovisceral reflex affecting the lungs.

The liver is responsible for a number of metabolic functions, which include the metabolism of ingested fats and proteins, the storage and release of carbohydrates, the synthesis and degradation of cholesterol and hormones, and the detoxification of drugs and toxins. The liver also transforms a chemical called bilirubin into a form that can be safely excreted from the body and is responsible for the synthesis of clotting factors.

Any impairment in the metabolism of protein, carbohydrate, or fat can be devastating. When the detoxification function of the liver is impaired, toxins build up in the body and can cause illness or even death. One of the earliest signs of a buildup of toxins from liver failure is a yellow coloring of the skin and eyes due to a buildup of bilirubin. Very high levels of bilirubin can cause permanent neurological damage. When the liver does not produce clotting factors, dangerous bleeding episodes become common.

Decreased blood flow to the liver has been shown to result in increased bilirubin levels, decreased clotting factors, and impairment in the metabolic and detoxification functions.[7] These effects can lead to metabolic disturbances, neurological damage, and uncontrolled bleeding. Decreased blood perfusion of the liver can also cause cholecystitis and pancreatitis.[8] Cholecystitis is an acute inflammation of the gall bladder, which can cause nausea, vomiting, and pain. Pancreatitis, an acute inflammation of the pancreas caused by the release of pancreatic enzymes, can cause severe pain and is often fatal. Many of these effects of decreased blood profusion to the liver are delayed and can cause illness, or even death, days after an attack.

The liver can be attacked with an aberrant reference combination facilitating the T6–7 levels of the spinal cord. The attack must include an additional point that can facilitate the sympathetic nerves of the liver because the intestines connect to the spinal cord at the same level. Striking the organ trauma point can directly damage the liver or the membranous capsule around the liver. Damage to either will stimulate the sympathetic nerves of the liver.

The kidneys are responsible for controlling the balance of fluid and electrolytes (sodium, potassium, and phosphate) in the body. In response to a decrease in circulating red blood cells, the kidneys produce a chemical called erythropoietin, which signals the bone marrow to produce new red blood cells. In addition, the kidneys convert vitamin D to its active form, which causes increased calcium absorption from the digestive tract and decreased calcium loss from bones.

Decreased blood perfusion of the kidneys can cause acute renal failure, leading to disturbances in fluid and electrolytes.

This can result in heart failure from fluid overload, cardiac arrest from abnormal potassium levels, and seizures from abnormal sodium levels. A chronic decrease in the blood perfusion of the kidneys can cause chronic renal failure. This can lead to deficiencies in erythropoietin and the active form of vitamin D, which can cause anemia (a decrease in red blood cells that can lead to shortness of breath, dizziness, and heart attack) and osteomalcia (a softening of the bones that can lead to deformities and fractures).

As with the liver, the kidneys will only be affected by an aberrant reference combination if the organ trauma point was also attacked to facilitate the sympathetic nerves. The reason for this is that the T10–11 levels of the spinal cord are also connected to the sympathetic nerves of the intestines, colon, and genitals.

The digestive tract is responsible for absorbing nutrients and water from ingested substances. A decrease in the blood perfusion of the digestive tract can lead to many complications, including stress ulcers and an ileus, which is a complete lack of intestinal motility.[9] The symptoms of an ulcer include pain, nausea, and vomiting. Associated complications include perforation, which can lead to fatal hemorrhaging unless treated surgically, and occult blood loss, which can lead to anemia or shock. The symptoms of an ileus include pain, distention, and vomiting. An ileus can also lead to intestinal perforation with hemorrhaging. A chronic decrease in blood flow to the digestive tract can cause an array of digestive disturbances including nausea, vomiting, and malabsorbtion.

The digestive system is also very sensitive to changes in the balance between the sympathetic and parasympathetic nervous systems. Increased sympathetic stimulation can lead to constipation, bloating, and abdominal pain. In addition, recent research has found that it can disrupt the mucosal protective layer of the digestive tract, leading to an increased incidence of ulcers.[10] Increased parasympathetic stimulation of the digestive tract can cause vomiting, diarrhea, and abdominal cramps.

The digestive tract can be attacked with an aberrant reference combination facilitating the T6–L2 levels of the spinal cord. Altering the balance between the sympathetic and parasympathetic nervous systems can also affect the digestive tract. Because the digestive system is so sensitive to changes in the autonomic nervous system, almost any dim-mak point can affect it.

There are additional methods of disrupting the blood flow to the internal organs. The blood perfusion of an internal organ can be completely cut off when a blood clot or a piece of artherosclerotic plaque occludes one of its major blood vessels. *Embolus* is the medical term for a blood clot or a piece of plaque traveling in the blood stream. When an embolus lodges in a blood vessel that is too small to allow passage, a complete blockage of the vessel occurs. This often occurs naturally in the arteries supplying the brain, heart, and digestive tract (mesenteric circulation). Interestingly, striking certain dim-mak points can also cause this effect.

Striking the points located over the carotid arteries in an older person can cause a stroke because the carotid arteries are prone to plaque formation, which increases with age. When a piece of this plaque enters the cerebral circulation, it can lodge in a small blood vessel and occlude it. This can result in a stroke because a portion of the brain will be deprived of blood. The greatest buildup of plaque occurs at the bifurcation of the carotid arteries.[11] This location coincides with the Stomach 9 point. Thus, striking this point can cause a piece of plaque to break off and occlude one of the cerebral blood vessels resulting in a stroke and/or death. Furthermore, a strike to the Stomach 9 point can cause a plaque to weaken. This can result in a piece breaking off at a later date and thus cause a stroke and/or death some time after the initial attack.

Another method of disrupting the blood flow to the brain

involves head trauma. One of the most lethal complications of head trauma is an epidural hematoma, which is a collection of blood between the skull and brain. This can cause dizziness, delirium, neurological deficits, and usually death if untreated. One of the unique clinical features of an epidural hematoma is that after the initial effects of the trauma patients will usually have an interval where they are completely lucid. This is then followed by a rapid deterioration in mental status, coma, and death. The most common cause of an epidural hematoma is direct trauma to the temporal bone resulting in a fracture, which can tear the middle meningeal artery.[12] This can be explained by the fact that this artery lies directly beneath the temporal bone, which is one of the weakest areas of the skull.

It is actually quite difficult to fracture any of the skull bones because it requires a great deal of force. However, this is not the case with the sutures of the skull bones. Sutures are areas where the skull bones interlock with each other. They are actually composed of small interlocking pieces of bone. Interestingly, some of the most deadly dim-mak points are located directly over the sutures of the temporal bone. Thus, a powerful attack to one of these points can fracture the temporal bone and cause a tear in the middle meningeal artery, leading to an epidural hematoma and death. The points are Gall Bladder 4, Gall Bladder 5, and Stomach 8. The Gall Bladder 5 point is the most dangerous because it is located directly over a major branch of the middle meningeal artery and a weak suture called the pterion. Because the pterion is actually composed of two sutures, it is much weaker than the other sutures of the temporal bone.

All three of these points are also located over branches of the auriculotemporal nerve. This is significant because this nerve is actually a branch of the facial nerve. Thus, these points can also cause a vasovagal faint or cardiac arrest. In addition, because a person with an epidural hematoma could have a lucid interval followed by coma and death, these points could be related to the legend of a delayed death touch.

Striking points on the legs can cause a pulmonary embolism. The effects of this disorder include decreased blood pressure, lung damage, circulatory collapse, and death.[13] The most common cause of a pulmonary embolism is a blood clot that formed in the leg veins and migrated to the pulmonary arteries. Thus, any time there is a blood clot in one of the leg veins there is a risk of a pulmonary embolism. There are three major risk factors for developing blood clots in the leg veins: immobility, injury, and an inherent tendency to form blood clots. Additionally, it has been found that external leg trauma can cause a blood clot to form in one of the leg veins.[14] This is significant because some of the dim-mak points are located on vulnerable portions of the major leg veins. Thus, striking one of these points can cause a blood clot to form in a leg vein, which can migrate to one of the pulmonary arteries and cause a pulmonary embolism. Furthermore, a very strong attack on one of these points can result in immobilization of the injured leg, which will further increase the likelihood of a pulmonary embolism. A person with a tendency to form blood clots would be even more vulnerable to such an attack. If such a person had preexisting blood clots in the leg veins, a strike could knock one of them loose, resulting a pulmonary embolism. This brings us to the last aspect of attacking the leg veins: a blood clot in a leg vein might cause a pulmonary embolism instantly, or it might stay in the vein and cause a pulmonary embolism at a later date. This is interesting because it shows how an attack to the leg points can cause a delayed death.

The internal organs can also be attacked directly through the organ trauma points. These points are located on vulnerable portions of the internal organs, and attacking them can cause organ failure, a vasovagal faint, or rupture of the organ leading to internal hemorrhaging and death. All of the internal organs have an extensive blood supply that causes them to bleed profusely when injured. Consequently, a person can quickly bleed to death from a ruptured organ. Since an increase in blood pressure and heart rate can cause a ruptured organ to bleed even more profusely, these points are potentiated by increased activity of the sympathetic nervous system. All of the internal organs located in the abdomen can be attacked in this manner, but the spleen is the easiest organ to rupture.

The spleen is located on the left side of the body just under the eighth and ninth ribs. A very strong attack to this area can fracture the ribs and damage the spleen. In some cases, striking up under the front of the left ribs can also cause trauma to the spleen. The spleen contains a large amount of blood and is enveloped in a membranous capsule. When the spleen is ruptured, this capsule can control the bleeding for a short period of time. Because of this, a person can have a ruptured spleen and be without symptoms for a number of days. Eventually the capsule will burst, resulting in uncontrolled bleeding. When this occurs, there will be a sudden drop in blood pressure leading to a loss of consciousness, shock, and death.

In conclusion, attacking the internal organs through the dim-mak points can cause extensive damage that can be explained by medical science. The effects of attacking an organ include a loss of consciousness, organ failure, and death due to hemorrhage. The rate of organ failure depends on the organ as well as the method of attack. Combining a vasovagal faint with a somatovisceral reflex can cause a drastic reduction in the blood perfusion of an internal organ, resulting in extensive damage. Attacking the carotid arteries can cause a piece of arthrosclerotic plaque to break off and cause a stroke or death. Attacking the points on the temporal bone can cause a tear in the middle meningeal artery, leading to an epidural hematoma and death. Attacking certain leg points can cause a blood clot in a leg vein, which can travel to the lungs and cause a pulmonary embolism. Finally, some of the internal organs can be attacked directly through the organ trauma points. Striking these points can cause lethal hemorrhaging, especially if the sympathetic nervous system was stimulated prior to the attack. Because they can have delayed effects, it is conceivable that these methods could be related to the origin of the delayed death touch legend.

Chapter 7

The Heart

I t should come as no surprise that dim-mak's most lethal effects involve the heart. The fact that sudden cardiac death can be caused by abnormalities in the autonomic nervous system provides a clue to unlocking the mystery of dim-mak's lethal effects. The study of modern neurocardiology provides evidence that many dim-mak points are actually neurologically connected to the heart. Stimulating these points can adversely affect the autonomic control of the heart, leading to sudden cardiac death. In addition, attacking certain points on the chest can cause direct cardiac trauma, which has also been linked to sudden cardiac death. This chapter will explore the basic neurocardiology related to dim-mak, the pathophysiology of attacking the heart points, and the dim-mak mechanisms of causing sudden cardiac death.

All of the points can have an effect on the heart in one way or another. It is this aspect of dim-mak that makes all of the points dangerous. The cardiac effects of increased sympathetic stimulation will be discussed first because almost all of the points can increase the activity of the sympathetic nervous system. Increased sympathetic stimulation of the heart increases the cardiac output and enables the heart to deliver more oxygenated blood to working muscles. Although this is a normal response to exercise or a threat, excessive sympathetic stimulation of the heart can be dangerous.

The sympathetic nervous system accelerates the rate at which an electrical current will distribute across the heart muscle, causing it to beat faster and pump harder. This causes the heart muscle to require more blood because it requires more oxygen. The coronary arteries are usually able to supply adequate blood flow to cover the increased oxygen demand. However, stimulation of the sympathetic nervous system can cause a spasm of the coronary arteries.[1] The coronary blood flow is then decreased. The combination of increased oxygen demand and decreased coronary blood flow leads to a state of oxygen deprivation, which can cause symptoms of angina and cardiac damage. This type of angina is actually called prinzmetal's variant angina.[2] When a severe spasm totally occludes part of the coronary blood flow, a section of the heart dies and the individual suffers a heart attack. Thus, a severe coronary artery spasm can actually cause a heart attack.[3] This is actually more common than one would like to believe. In up to 10 percent of heart attack victims, there is no evidence of a thrombus (blood clot) or artherosclerotic disease in the coronary blood vessels.[4] Consequently, in these patients, the heart attack is most likely due to a spasm of the coronary arteries.

In older individuals and those with heart disease, even small increases in the sympathetic stimulation of the heart can be fatal. The reason for this is that these individuals have an increased incidence of atherosclerosis. A coronary artery spasm at the site of an artherosclerotic plaque can precipitate a heart attack.[5] The artherosclerosis causes narrowing of the coronary arteries and, consequently, decreased blood flow to the heart. When the blood flow is reduced further by a coronary artery spasm, the heart is further deprived of blood, resulting in a heart attack.

Increased sympathetic stimulation of the heart can also cause abnormalities in the heart's electrical conduction system, leading to abnormal heart rhythms called arrhythmias. There are many different types of arrhythmias. Some are benign with a good prognosis and others are lethal. Arrhythmias will be covered in detail later in this chapter. For now, it is important for one to know that increased sympathetic stimulation of the heart is associated with an increased incidence of arrhythmias.

There are two different ways in which the dim-mak points can affect the sympathetic stimulation of the heart. The first involves pain. As stated in Chapter 2, a somatosympathetic reflex is a pain-induced increase in the activity of the sympathetic nervous system. This usually causes an increase in heart rate and blood pressure, but in an individual with heart disease, it can precipitate a heart attack or a fatal arrhythmia. Since almost all of the points can cause pain, this is the easiest method of increasing the sympathetic stimulation of the heart. It is also why stimulation of any of the points can be dangerous in an individual with heart disease.

The second method of increasing the sympathetic stimulation of the heart involves nerves that are neurologically connected to the cardiac sympathetic nerves through convergence. There is scientific evidence that these nerves can directly stimulate the cardiac sympathetic nerves.[6] Thus, attacking the points on these nerves can directly increase the sympathetic stimulation of the heart. This is significant because medical research has found that direct stimulation of the cardiac sympathetic nerves can lead to arrhythmias.[7] These arrhythmias include supraventricular tachycardia with fainting and ventricular fibrillation with death. This second method increases the sympathetic stimulation of the heart much more than a somatosympathetic reflex. Consequently, attacking the points on these nerves is much more likely to cause an arrhythmia or a heart attack, even in a healthy individual.

The ulnar nerve, the median nerve, the first five dorsal nerve roots, and the first five intercostal nerves all have a direct neurological connection to the cardiac sympathetic nerves. Thus, attacking the points on these nerves can directly stimulate the cardiac sympathetic nerves. The first five dorsal nerve roots are located under the Bladder 11-15 points. The ulnar nerve can be attacked through the heart points on the arm, and the median nerve can be attacked through the pericardial points on the arm. The first five intercostal nerves can be attacked through Conception Vessel 17-20, Kidney 22-26, Stomach 15-17, Gall Bladder 22 and 23, Spleen 17, Lung 1 and 2, and Pericardium 1. The arrhythmia point[8] is located in the right fifth intercostal space at the Kidney 22 point and is actually located on a cutaneous branch of the fifth intercostal nerve. Pain in this nerve has been linked to a supraventricular tachycardia (fast irregular heartbeat) that resolves when the pain is alleviated.[9] There are two additional points that can increase the sympathetic stimulation of the heart. The left stellate sympathetic ganglion can be attacked through the Large Intestine 17 point, and the left superior cervical sympathetic ganglion can be attacked through the Small Intestine 17 point. All of these points will be referred to as the sympathetic heart points. (See Figure 18.) It is important to understand which points increase the sympathetic stimulation of the heart because, in addition to causing a heart attack or arrhythmia, they can be used as set-up points.

The other method of affecting the autonomic control of the heart involves attacking points that can increase the parasympathetic stimulation of the heart. The parasympathetic effects on the heart include a slowing of the heart's electrical conduction system and a decrease in heart rate. This leads to a slower heartbeat with softer contractions. Excessive increases in the parasympathetic effects on the heart can cause heart block, a loss of consciousness, and cardiac arrest.

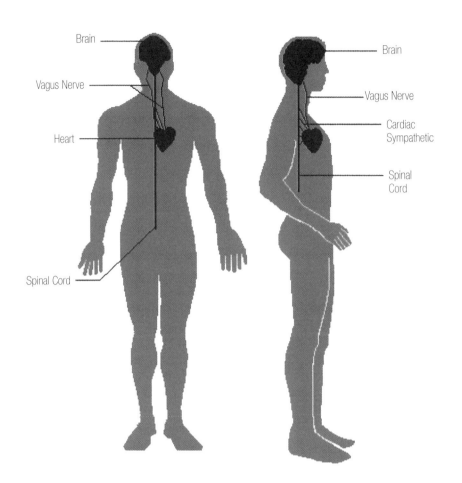

FIGURE 20
The cardiac autonomic nerves.

All of the parasympathetic effects on the heart occur through the vagus nerve. This is the only nerve that can increase the parasympathetic effects on the heart directly. The cranial and occipital nerves, the carotid sinus, and aberrant reference all increase the parasympathetic effects on the heart by stimulating an area of the brain connected to the vagus nerve. This area, called the nucleus tractus solitarii, is responsible for causing a vasovagal faint in addition to increasing the parasympathetic effects on the heart. Thus, there is always the possibility of causing a vasovagal faint when the parasympathetic effects on the heart are increased.

The vagus nerve runs down both sides of the neck and has branches that connect directly to the heart and to most of the other internal organs (see fig. 20). Medical research has shown that excessive stimulation of the vagus nerve can cause arrhythmias and cardiac arrest.[10] The left side vagus nerve terminates in an area of the heart called the atrio-ventricular node. Excessive parasympathetic activity in this area can cause heart block, which is a slowing or a complete interruption of the electrical conduction from the atria to the ventricles. Heart block can result in fainting or death. The right side vagus nerve terminates in an area called the sino-atrial node. Excessive parasympathetic stimulation of this node can cause the heart to beat very slowly or even stop, resulting in cardiac arrest. This can also result in fainting or even death. Cardiac arrest is much more likely to occur when the vagus nerve is stimulated on both sides simultaneously because the effect on the heart is exaggerated.

The dim-mak points that stimulate the parasympathetic effects on the heart include Stomach 9; Gall Bladder 1–6 and 13–18; Stomach 2, 3, and 5–7; Bladder 6–8; Triple Warmer 17 and 23; and Small Intestine 16 and 18. The vagus nerve also has branches on the neck that connect directly to the heart. One of these, the superior cervical cardiac vagal nerve, is vulnerable to attack under the Stomach 10 point. All of these points will be referred to as the parasympathetic heart points. (See Figures 9 and 17.) Because these points increase the parasympathetic effects on the heart, they can cause a knockout or cardiac arrest. However, in order to cause cardiac arrest, the attack must be powerful enough to cause very strong parasympathetic effects on the heart. This can be accomplished by combining these points, using set-up points, or combining both of these methods. An understanding of how to increase the parasympathetic effects on the heart is essential for two reasons. First, all of the methods of increasing the parasympathetic effects on the heart are synergistic when used together. Second, increased parasympathetic effects on the heart can set up certain heart points on the chest to cause cardiac arrest.

CARDIAC ARRHYTHMIAS

The most common cause of death during a heart attack is not damaged cardiac tissue, but rather a fatal arrhythmia. An arrhythmia is an abnormal rhythm of heartbeats. Some arrhythmias can cause fainting with chest pain, and others can cause death. The heartbeat normally has a regular, steady rhythm. However, the sympathetic and parasympathetic nervous systems can change this rhythm. There is a large body of evidence suggesting that the actual cause of most fatal arrhythmias is an imbalance between the sympathetic and parasympathetic influences on the heart.[11] Interestingly, attacking the dim-mak points can directly alter this balance.

Attacking the points that increase the activity of the sympathetic nervous system can cause death due to an arrhythmia called ventricular fibrillation. It has been found that excessive sympathetic stimulation can increase the vulnerability of the heart to this type of arrhythmia.[12] Thus, there is a chance of causing ventricular fibrillation whenever the sympathetic heart points are attacked. In addition, research has shown that an imbalance in the activity of the right and left cardiac sympathetic nerves can also lead to an arrhythmia.[13] One would be inclined to think that attacking the sympathetic heart points on only one side would cause such an imbalance. This is correct but only if the left-side cardiac sympathetic nerves are stimulated. Medical research has found that when the left-side cardiac sympathetic nerves are stimulated alone, they are more likely to cause an arrhythmia.[14] Perhaps this is the reason many of the traditional forms contain more attacks with the right hand.

Certain points on the chest can be used to attack the heart directly. There are numerous medical reports of sudden death caused by chest wall trauma. The medical term for this phenomenon is *commotio cordis*, which is Latin for heart concussion. Reported cases include trauma from baseballs, hockey pucks, hockey sticks, knees, shoulders, punches, and karate kicks.[15, 16, 17, 18] The autopsies of these cases revealed no other cause of death, and the only evidence of trauma was a contusion on the chest.[19] All of the cases had trauma to the same areas of the chest, and the most common areas correlated with the Stomach 18, Kidney 22, Kidney 23, and Kidney 24 points on the left side of the chest. From this point forward, these points will be referred to as the autonomic heart points.

Recently, medical science has found that the mechanism of commotio cordis involves vulnerable periods of electrical activity in the heart.[20] It was found that there is a vulnerable period when the heart resets its electrical system after a beat. An impact to the chest wall during this interval was found to cause ventricular fibrillation.[21] An impact to the chest wall during the actual electrical conduction through the heart was found to cause heart block and cardiac arrest.[22] In this research, the area of impact was located directly over the left ventricle.[23] This area correlates with the autonomic heart points.

The autonomic heart points can cause two different effects depending on which points are used as a setup. This is why these points are almost always used for a final attack. In many of the traditional forms, a strike to the chest follows numerous techniques. This strike is attacking the autonomic heart points after first stimulating the sympathetic or parasympathetic nervous systems. As previously stated, ventricular fibrillation has been found to be much more frequent when there is a high level of sympathetic nervous system activity. Increased sympathetic stimulation results in a faster conduction of the heart's electrical system. This means that the conduction period is much shorter than the repolarizing period. Thus, there is a greater chance that a strike to the heart will occur when the electrical system is repolarizing. In other words, when the sympathetic effects on the heart are increased, there is a greater likelihood of chest trauma causing ventricular fibrillation. Consequently, attacking the sympathetic heart points will increase cardiac sympathetic stimulation and set up the autonomic heart points to cause ventricular fibrillation and death.

Conversely, when the parasympathetic effects on the heart are increased, the electrical conduction slows down. This means that there is a greater likelihood that a strike to the chest will occur during the actual conduction of electricity though the heart. Thus, when the parasympathetic effects on the heart are increased, there is a greater likelihood of chest trauma causing heart block or cardiac arrest. One can increase the parasympathetic effects on the heart by attacking the parasympathetic heart points or by using an aberrant reference technique. The autonomic heart points will then be set up to cause heart block and cardiac arrest.

One might question how striking the chest can generate enough force to actually cause heart trauma. The answer to this question is fairly straightforward. The rib cage actually has a great deal of elasticity. Anyone who has ever performed or observed CPR can attest to this fact. During CPR, the ribs are actually compressed, causing the heart to be squeezed between the sternum and spinal column. This forces blood out of the heart to the rest of the body. Because of the rib cage pliability, it does not take a great deal of force to compress the heart. If a similar movement were performed quickly, it could easily traumatize the heart. Thus, a quick, powerful thrust against the autonomic heart points could compress the sternum and injure the heart. The evidence that such a blow can cause heart trauma can be found in the case reports of commotio cordis. In most cases, the force of the blow was relatively modest.[24]

In one experiment on commotio cordis, a small wooden object the size and weight of a baseball was thrust at the chest of experimental animals at a velocity of 30 mph.[25] This consistently produced cardiac arrest and ventricular fibrillation.[26] Most proficient martial artists can deliver a blow with a velocity much greater than 30 mph, and the use of the hips allows one to place a larger amount of mass behind the strike. Thus, it is conceivable that a well-trained martial artist could deliver an impact equal to or greater than that used in the study.

SYNERGISTIC COMBINATIONS

Many of the heart points can be combined for a synergistic effect. For example, an attack to the heart or pericardial points on the arm can increase the sympathetic stimulation of the heart. Since multiple methods of increasing the sympathetic stimulation of the heart are synergistic because of summation, one could follow this with an attack to the heart points on the chest or back. This would magnify the sympathetic stimulation of the heart. If an attack to the heart or pericardial points on the arm was followed by an attack to the head or neck points, the parasympathetic stimulation of the heart would be magnified. This occurs because increased sympathetic stimulation magnifies the parasympathetic effects on the heart.[27] As a general rule, after the sympathetic heart points are attacked, the other sympathetic heart points, the parasympathetic heart points, and the autonomic heart points all become more effective.

It should be noted that there is one particular combination of heart points that will not be synergistic. The sympathetic heart points can reverse the effects of the parasympathetic heart points. Consequently, the sympathetic heart points can only be attacked before the parasympathetic heart points. If they are attacked after the parasympathetic heart points, they will negate the parasympathetic effects on the heart. Thus, after attacking points on the head and neck, one can only attack other head and neck points, the Conception Vessel 14 point, the autonomic heart points, or an aberrant reference combination.

In summary, the heart can be attacked in four ways. First, the points that increase the sympathetic effects on the heart can be attacked to cause an arrhythmia or a heart attack. Second, the points that increase the parasympathetic effects on the heart can be attacked to cause a vasovagal faint or cardiac arrest. Third, the autonomic heart points on the chest can be attacked after the sympathetic effects on the heart are increased to cause ventricular fibrillation. Fourth, the autonomic heart points can be attacked after the parasympathetic effects on the heart are increased to cause cardiac arrest. Additionally, there are three basic methods of synergistically combining the heart points: the sympathetic heart points can be combined, the parasympathetic heart points can be combined, and the parasympathetic heart points can be set up by the sympathetic heart points. If one were to keep these seven concepts in mind when analyzing the traditional forms, it would quickly become apparent that many of the techniques actually attack the heart points and are in fact, quite lethal.

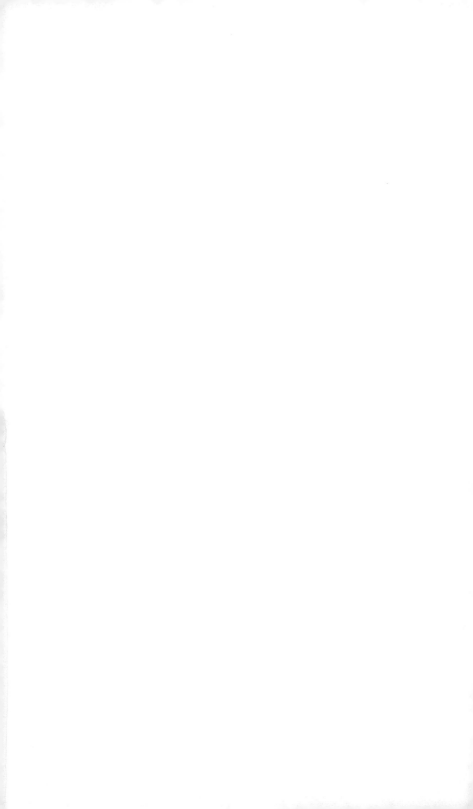

Chapter 8

Putting It All Together
The Basics

In the previous chapters, the important medical
concepts related to dim-mak were explained and
discussed in detail. The application of these concepts to the study of dim-mak increases the art's
credibility by providing a modern scientific explanation for its effects. In addition, the application of
medical science to dim-mak is useful when attempting to find and understand the dim-mak applications of the traditional forms. The latter requires a
firm grasp on the medical concepts in this book as
well as a strong foundation in the basic components
of dim-mak. With such tools, the martial artist can
analyze the traditional forms of his or her style for
potential dim-mak applications. This chapter provides a basic foundation that will enable the reader
to apply the concepts in this book to the study of
dim-mak. Before embarking on such a task, a clear
understanding of the medical concepts presented in
this book is essential. They are outlined here in a
simplified manner. A review of the previous chapters, if necessary, will provide a more in-depth
understanding of these concepts.

KEY CONCEPTS

Parasympathetic Nervous System—The part of the nervous system responsible for increasing the activity of the gastrointestinal system as well as decreasing the heart rate and blood pressure. Excessive activity can lead to diarrhea, vomiting, abdominal cramps, a vasovagal faint, and cardiac arrest.

Sympathetic Nervous System—The part of the nervous system responsible for increasing the heart rate, increasing the blood pressure, and decreasing the activity of the gastrointestinal system. Increased activity leads to many changes that prepare the individual for a confrontation. Some have called this the "fight or flight response." Excessive activity can lead to constipation, anxiety, arrhythmias, and a heart attack.

Vasovagal Faint—A medical term for loss of consciousness resulting from an increase in the parasympathetic effects on the heart and a concomitant decrease in the sympathetic effects on the blood vessels. Any technique that causes a vasovagal faint also has the potential to cause cardiac arrest because of the increased parasympathetic activity.

Vasovagal Points—The points that increase the parasympathetic effects on the heart and can cause a vasovagal faint (knockout), also known as the parasympathetic heart points (see figs. 9 and 17).

- *Cranial Nerves*—Gall Bladder 1–6, 13–18, Stomach 2, 3, Bladder 6–8, Triple Warmer 17 and 23, Small Intestine 17 and 18, Stomach 5–8, and Stomach 10 (vagal cardiac nerve).
  - Occipital nerves—Bladder 10, Gall Bladder 20
  - Carotid sinus—Stomach 9 point
  - Celiac plexus—Conception Vessel 14 point
  - Oculocardiac reflex—the eyeball

- *Aberrant Reference*—Pain coming from the heart, lung, digestive tract, bladder, and genitals.

All of the above have the ability to cause nausea, dizziness, fainting, and cardiac arrest.

Combination Points—The points that can affect multiple organs because they are connected to levels of the spinal cord that are connected to more than one internal organ: Lung 1–2; Stomach 15–17; Conception Vessel 14, 17–20; Kidney 23–26; Badder 11–14; Gall Bladder 22–23; Spleen 17; and Pericardium 4 (see fig. 10).

Aberrant Reference—The phenomenon whereby pain in two or more nerves on opposite sides of the body can cause pain in one of the internal organs that is connected to the spinal cord in the middle of where the two nerves connect. If the pain was in the heart, lung, digestive tract, bladder, or kidneys, it could result in a vasovagal faint or cardiac arrest caused by increased parasympathetic effects.

Convergence—The neurological connection between the sympathetic nerves from the internal organs and the external nerves of the body.

Facilitation—Stimulation of nerves, either directly or by aberrant reference, causes the spinal cord to become hypersensitive to further stimuli. This causes the other nerves connected to the hypersensitive spinal segment to have a magnified effect.

Somatovisceral Reflex—A decrease in blood flow to an organ caused by stimulation of nerves connected to that organ by convergence. A somatovisceral reflex affecting the heart can cause a heart attack. A somatovisceral reflex affecting the other internal organs can result in organ dysfunction or failure.

Summation—The additive effects of stimulating multiple nerves that affect the same section of the nervous system.

EFFECTS OF THE POINTS ON SPECIFIC ORGANS

For simplicity, the effects of the points on the major organs will be dealt with separately. The martial artist should bear in mind that attacking the nervous system will always affect the heart to some degree. Thus, any point can be lethal in an individual with heart disease. Even striking the stomach or intestines can cause a visceral type of pain that can lead to a vasovagal faint or cardiac arrest.

The Heart

The heart is the major organ affected by the dim-mak points. Increasing the parasympathetic effects will slow the heart rate and can cause a vasovagal faint, heart block, or cardiac arrest. Increasing the sympathetic stimulation of the heart enhances the parasympathetic effects on the heart and can cause a fatal arrhythmia or a heart attack. Stimulation of the direct points, the indirect points, and the use of aberrant reference can all cause a somatovisceral reflex, which can result in a vasovagal faint or a heart attack. The autonomic heart points will cause different effects depending on whether they follow the parasympathetic heart points or the sympathetic heart points.

Direct Heart Points
These points affect the heart directly:
- Heart and pericardial points on the arm, Stomach 18, Kidney 22 and 23, the vasovagal points, and Conception Vessel 14 and 17.
- The parasympathetic, sympathetic, and autonomic heart points.

Indirect Heart Points
These points will affect the heart only if first facilitated by stimulation of the direct heart points:

- The Bladder 11–14 points on the first four dorsal nerve roots.
- The points on the front of the torso that connect to the first five intercostal nerves: Stomach 15–17, Kidney 22–26, Conception Vessel 14, 17–20, Lung 1–2, Gall Bladder 22–23, Spleen 17, and Pericardium 4.

Parasympathetic Heart Points

These points directly increase the parasympathetic effects on the heart and are the same as the vasovagal points (see figs. 9 and 17):

- Cranial nerves—Gall Bladder 1–6, 3–18; Stomach 2, 3; Bladder 6–8; Triple Warmer 17 and 23; Small Intestine 17 and 18; Stomach 5–8; and Stomach 10 (vagal cardiac nerve).
- Occipital nerves—Bladder 10, Gall Bladder 20.
- Carotid sinus—Stomach 9.
- Celiac plexus—Conception Vessel 14.
- Oculocardiac reflex—the eyeball.

Sympathetic Heart Points

These points can directly increase the sympathetic stimulation of the heart (see figs. 10 and 18):

- Any point that causes pain.
- Conception Vessel 17, Kidney 22 and 23, Stomach 16–18, Pericardium 1, Lung 1–2, Bladder 11–15, Small Intestine 17, Gall Bladder 22–23, Spleen 17, and the heart and pericardial points on the arm.

Autonomic Heart Points

These points can cause cardiac arrest if the parasympathetic effects on the heart are increased and a fatal arrhythmia if the sympathetic stimulation of the heart is increased (see fig. 19): Stomach 18, Kidney 22, and Kidney 23 on the left side of the chest.

Aberrant Reference

Use of the following can facilitate the T1–5 levels of the spinal cord and affect the heart by causing a somatovisceral reflex. Because T1-4 can also affect the lungs, one must stimulate the heart or pericardial points on the arm nerves for these combinations to register at the heart.

- Stimulation of the heart or pericardial points on the ulnar or median nerve in combination with the following: Lung 1–2, Stomach 15–18, Kidney 22–26, Pericardium 1, Liver 13 and 14, Gall Bladder 22–24, Spleen 17 and 21, and Conception Vessel 14–20.
- Stimulation of the arm points on the ulnar and radial nerves in combination with any of the point combinations involving the ulnar nerve; Conception Vessel 6, Gall Bladder 25, Bladder 23, Spleen 12, or Liver 12.

Heart Attack Points

Stimulation of the following points can induce a heart attack through either somatovisceral reflexes or sympathetic stimulation of the heart:

- Any of the direct or indirect heart points after they have been facilitated.
- All of the aberrant reference combinations that can cause facilitation of T1–5.

The Lungs

The sympathetic nerves connected to lungs and airways can cause a vasovagal faint or cardiac arrest when stimulated. They can be attacked through the direct points, the indirect points, or an aberrant reference combination. Increasing the sympathetic stimulation of the lungs will cause the airways to open. This is not harmful. Increasing the parasympathetic effects on the lungs will cause the airways to close, resulting in difficulty breathing, but this is not possible with the dim-mak points. Thus, the dim-mak points can only affect the lungs through direct trauma or a somatovisceral reflex.

Methods of Attacking the Lungs

Stimulation of the first 10 intercostal nerves can cause the intercostal muscles to spasm, causing an inability to breathe in the recipient of the attack. The points are Stomach 16–18, Kidney 22–26, Conception Vessel 14, 17–20, Lung 1–2, Pericardium 4, Liver 13 and 14, Gall Bladder 22–24, and Spleen 17 and 21 (see fig. 10).

Stimulation of the phrenic nerve or the celiac plexus can cause a spasm of the diaphragm. This will also cause the recipient of the attack to feel as though he or she cannot breathe. The phrenic nerve is located under the Large Intestine 17 point, and the celiac plexus is located under the Conception Vessel 14 point (see figs. 9 and 10).

Direct Lung Points

The following can stimulate the sympathetic nerves of the lung, which can cause a vasovagal faint, a somatovisceral reflex, or cardiac arrest due to increased parasympathetic effects on the heart: the points on the radial nerve, including Large Intestine 4–14, Lung 5–8, and Triple Warmer 11 and 12; and the phrenic nerve under Large Intestine 17 (see figs. 10 and 11).

Indirect Lung Points

These points only affect the lung when the T1–4 levels of the spinal cord are facilitated by prior stimulation of the radial nerve (see figs. 10 and 11):

- The Bladder 11–14 points on the first four dorsal nerve roots.
- The points on the first four intercostal nerves: Lung 1–2, Stomach 15–17, Kidney 23–26, Conception Vessel 17–20, Gall Bladder 22, Spleen 17, and Pericardium 4.

Aberrant Reference

The following will facilitate the T1–4 levels of the spinal cord and can cause a somatovisceral reflex affecting the lungs in addition to a vasovagal faint. Because the T1–4 spinal levels can also affect the heart, these combinations will only affect the lungs when the radial nerve is stimulated. If the ulnar or median nerves were stimulated, these combinations would affect the heart.

- Stimulation of the lung, large intestine, or triple warmer points on the arm in combination with Liver 12–14; Gall Bladder 22 and 24–25; Spleen 12, 17, and 21; Conception Vessel 6, 14, and 17–20; Bladder 11–15 and 23; and Large Intestine 17 (phrenic nerve).
- Simultaneous striking of points on the front of the body that are horizontal or diagonal after stimulating the radial nerve: Stomach 15–18 and Kidney 22–26, bilaterally horizontal; Lung 1 in combination diagonally with Liver 14; and Gall Bladder 22–24, Spleen 21, or Conception Vessel 14.

The Gastrointestinal System

The gastrointestinal (GI) system consists of the stomach, large intestine, small intestine, gall bladder, and liver. Stimulation of a somatovisceral reflex can cause a number of digestive problems. Stimulation of sympathetic nerves connected to the digestive tract can cause a vasovagal faint, nausea, vomiting, dizziness, and possibly cardiac arrest. Increasing the sympathetic stimulation of the digestive tract can cause bloating, nausea, pain, and constipation. Increasing the parasympathetic stimulation of the digestive tract can cause vomiting, cramps, and diarrhea. The gastrointestinal system is normally attacked with aberrant reference combinations to cause a somatovisceral reflex or through the autonomic nervous system to cause dysfunction.

Direct GI Points

These points can affect the gastrointestinal system directly (see fig. 10): Bladder 16–20, Liver 13–14, Gall Bladder 24, Conception Vessel 14, and Spleen 21.

Organ Trauma Points

These points can cause direct trauma to the organs mentioned: Stomach 25 (intestines), Stomach 20 and 21 on the right (stomach), Conception Vessel 8–12 (intestines), Spleen 16 (liver), and Liver 13 (liver).

Direct Parasympathetic GI Points

These points can increase the parasympathetic effects on the gastrointestinal system:

- Any of the aberrant reference techniques affecting the GI system.
- Any point or combination that can cause a vasovagal faint.

Direct Sympathetic GI Points

These points can increase the sympathetic stimulation of the GI system (see fig. 10):

- The Bladder 16–20 points on the dorsal nerve roots.
- The 6th–10th intercostal nerves located at Liver 13 and 14, Gall Bladder 24, Conception Vessel 14, and Spleen 21.
- Any point that causes pain can increase the activity of the sympathetic nervous system due to a somatosympathetic reflex.

Aberrant Reference

The following combinations can facilitate the T6–10 levels of the spinal cord and can cause a vasovagal faint or somatovisceral reflex.

The heart and pericardial points on the arm will cause pain from the intestines if combined with Spleen 6 and 9–11; Gall Bladder 31, 39, and 41; Liver 3, 6, and 11; Kidney 6 and 8; Bladder 57, 60, 62, and 40; or Stomach 34, 36, 38, and 41.

The heart and pericardial points on the arm will cause pain from the stomach if combined with Spleen 12 or Liver 12.

The lung, large intestine, and triple warmer points on the arm will cause pain from the stomach if combined with

Spleen 6 and 9–12; Gall Bladder 31; Liver 6, 11, and 12; or Stomach 34.

The lung, large intestine, and triple warmer points on the arm will cause pain from the intestines if combined with Gall Bladder 41, Liver 3, or Stomach 36, 38, and 41.

The following will simplify using aberrant reference to attack the gastrointestinal system:

- The heart and pericardial points in combination with any of the opposite leg points will affect the intestines.
- The heart and pericardial points in combination with Spleen 12 or Liver 12 will affect the stomach.
- The points on the radial nerve (lung, large intestine, and triple warmer) in combination with the points on the foot will affect the intestines.
- The points on the radial nerve in combination with the points on the leg or groin will affect the stomach.

The Genitourinary System

The genitourinary (GU) system includes the genitals, bladder, and kidneys. The nerves innervating these organs are extremely sensitive. An attack to these nerves can cause a vasovagal faint as well as increased parasympathetic stimulation of the heart. If an attack did not cause a vasovagal faint, it would cause a great deal of pain with nausea and vomiting due to a reflex stimulation of the parasympathetic nervous system.

Direct GU Points

These points can directly affect the organs of the genitourinary system:

- The testicles are not points but they can be struck directly.
- The ovaries located under Spleen 13.
- The kidneys are located under Bladder 23 and 52.
- The bladder is under Conception Vessel 3–6.

Indirect GU Points

These points will affect the genitourinary system only

when the T11–L2 levels of the spinal cord are facilitated (see fig. 10): Liver 12, Gall Bladder 25, Liver 13, Spleen 11 and 12, and Bladder 21–24.

Aberrant Reference

These combinations facilitate the T10–L2 levels of the spinal cord and can cause a vasovagal faint or a somatovisceral reflex. There are no aberrant reference combinations using the arm nerves, but there are combinations of points on the body and legs, which will be covered in the advanced section.

APPLYING MEDICAL SCIENCE TO DIM-MAK

This text contains a great deal of information, and it might seem difficult to remember all the different effects of the points and nerves. The points can be simplified by grouping them according to their effects on the nervous and cardiovascular systems.

The points on the arm usually increase the sympathetic effects on all the organs. The heart points on the arm, chest, and back all increase the sympathetic stimulation of the heart (see figs. 10 and 11). The head and neck points increase the parasympathetic effects on all the organs, but the heart is the most affected (see fig. 9). With all the points, the heart is usually affected more than any other organ, especially when the heart points are stimulated. The only exceptions to these general rules are the Small Intestine 17, Large Intestine 17, and Conception Vessel 14 points. The Small Intestine 17 and Large Intestine 17 points can increase the sympathetic stimulation of the heart. The Conception Vessel 14 point will increase the parasympathetic effects on the gastrointestinal system unless it is combined with the heart points, which will cause it to increase the parasympathetic effects on the heart.

When the bladder points on the back are attacked, they directly increase the sympathetic stimulation of the internal organs. Some of these points will affect multiple organs because the sympathetic nerves from these organs overlap in the spinal cord. When such points are attacked, the other points used in combination will determine which organ is affected. The points on the body (i.e., chest, back, and abdomen) will usually cause a somatovisceral reflex as well as increased activity of the sympathetic nervous system. The organ that is affected by each point depends on convergence unless the point is used in combination with other points. Combinations of the arm points with the body or leg points will usually cause an aberrant reference effect, which increases the parasympathetic effects on the heart, leading to a vaso-vagal faint or cardiac arrest. However, an aberrant reference combination can also cause a somatovisceral reflex, leading to organ dysfunction or failure.

Learning the medical science behind dim-mak does not really change the martial artist's training until he or she reaches a very advanced level. Probably the oldest aspect of martial arts training involves kata practice. This is an essential element in the development of the martial artist as well as the person. Medical science does not change this fact. In the beginning, forms impart control, coordination, and balance in the martial artist. At the intermediate level, forms develop physical fitness and discipline. At the advanced level, the traditional forms train the mind so that attacking the dim-mak points becomes an automatic response requiring no conscious thought. This last level requires one to understand the dim-mak applications of the katas.

There are many dim-mak techniques contained within the traditional forms. The problem is finding them. The martial artist needs to open his or her mind and realize that any movement can be a dim-mak attack. This includes the set position of techniques as well as the blocking techniques. The angle and direction of each point will either stretch a nerve or compress it against a bone. Grappling moves will make use of the withdrawal reflex as well as reflex paralysis. Combinations of points should be synergistic based on summation, facilitation, and convergence.

Many opening moves of the traditional forms have dim-mak applications that attack the points on the arms. This seems reasonable because most confrontations start with some form of push, grab, or punch. It has been postulated that the arm points will set up many of the other points on the body to be more effective. Medical science supports this theory. At the most basic level, striking the arm will increase the activity of the sympathetic nervous system. This will enhance any technique that causes a vasovagal faint or increased parasympathetic activity. Attacking the arm points will also set up any other point that increases the activity of the sympathetic nervous system because of summation. In addition, increased sympathetic stimulation also potentiates the organ trauma points. At an advanced level, the arm points set up specific points on the body to become hypersensitive due to aberrant reference, facilitation, and convergence.

The angle and direction of attacking the points on the arm are usually toward oneself for the points on the inside of the arm and straight into the arm for the points on the outside of the arm. This practice can be shown to be effective based on medical science. A nerve sensing pain will be maximally stimulated when it is stretched, compressed against a bone, or both. Attacking the inner arm points toward oneself will stretch the arm nerves and compress them against the forearm bones. The points on the outer portion of the arm are only accessible in between the muscles and thus cannot be stretched when attacked. However, when these points are attacked straight into the arm, the radial nerve is compressed against the radius (bone).

The heart and pericardial points on the arm are known to affect the heart. Medical science has shown that these points have a direct neurological connection with the heart through the convergence of the median and ulnar nerves with the cardiac sympathetic nerves. Attacking these points can stimulate the cardiac sympathetic nerves, resulting in an increase in the sympathetic stimulation of the heart. The effects of this include a vasovagal faint, an arrhythmia, or a heart attack. In a healthy individual, usually only very intense stimulation of these nerves can produce such effects unless the points are used in combination with other points.

Attacking the radial nerve through the lung, large intestine, or triple warmer points can also cause a vasovagal faint. Here too, the stimulation of the nerve must be intense for such an effect to occur unless used in combination with other points. The effects of the radial nerve are explained by its neurological connection to the sympathetic nerves of the lung. Attacking the radial nerve can stimulate the sympathetic nerves, which will cause the brain to think that there was severe pain in the lungs and airways, resulting in a vasovagal faint.

There are two methods of increasing the stimulation of the arm nerves to the level required for serious effects. The first involves attacking multiple points on the same nerve, and the second involves attacking the points multiple times. Attacking multiple points on the same nerve will increase the stimulation of the nerve because of summation. Stimulating a nerve multiple times will increase the stimulation because there will be increased sensitivity in the nerve, the synapse, and the spinal cord with each attack. Consequently, when these points are attacked multiple times or in combination, there is a danger of causing very serious effects. In a confrontation, one could easily attack these points repeatedly during blocking or grabbing maneuvers. More importantly, one could inadvertently do so during practice.

The arm points are much more dangerous if they are followed by, or combined with, other synergistic points. The arm points can be synergistically combined with points on the head, neck, body, and legs. Attacking multiple points can increase the effectiveness of a technique. For example, one can increase the likelihood of causing a vasovagal faint by stimulating multiple vasovagal points. The vasovagal points will work synergistically to increase the stimulation of the nucleus tractus solitarii. In addition, the nucleus tractus solitarii can also be stimulated indirectly through the hypothalamus by attacking points that can cause severe pain. If the nucleus tractus solitarii were stimulated indirectly from nerve pain and directly from the vasovagal points, there would be a greater likelihood of causing a vasovagal faint and possibly cardiac arrest.

There are many methods of combining synergistic points to enhance the effects of an attack. As more synergistic points are added to a combination, the likelihood of causing serious effects increases in direct proportion. This brings us to the general rules about building combinations. Medical science is helpful in developing guidelines for finding and using synergistic combinations of points. At a basic level, these guidelines will allow one to understand how certain combinations of points work together. At an advanced level, one can use these guidelines to find the most lethal dim-mak combinations. Following are the basic guidelines for combining the dim-mak points:

- Any point or combination of points that increases the parasympathetic effects on the heart can be followed by, or used in combination with, any other point or combination that increases the parasympathetic effects on the heart. This includes the vasovagal points, which are the same as the parasympathetic heart points, and any aberrant reference combination affecting one of the internal organs.
- Any point or combination of points that increases the sympathetic stimulation of the heart can be followed by, or used in combination with, any other point or combination that increases the sympathetic stimulation of the heart.
- Any point or combination of points that increases the sympathetic stimulation of the heart can be followed by any point or combination of points that increases the parasympathetic effects on the heart.

- All of points that connect to the same level of the spinal cord can be used in combination or in sequence. This includes aberrant reference combinations because they facilitate specific levels of the spinal cord.
- The corresponding organ trauma or bladder point can follow an aberrant reference combination affecting an internal organ.

There are many applications of these guidelines. It would be impossible to list all of the possible combinations of points. Martial artists should analyze their forms to determine whether the dim-mak techniques follow these general rules. Let's look at combinations using the points on the arm to illustrate the application of these guidelines.

If the opposite leg nerves were attacked in combination with the ulnar or median nerve, the individual would feel pain in the intestines due to aberrant reference. This could cause abdominal cramps, diarrhea, and a vasovagal faint. Because this combination facilitates the T10–11 level of the spinal cord, one could follow this with an attack to any nerve connected to T10–11. This means that if the Bladder 20, Bladder 21, or Liver 13 points were attacked after this combination, there would be a greater chance of causing a vasovagal faint or cardiac arrest. In addition, because the effects of an aberrant reference combination result from an increase in the parasympathetic effects on the heart, one could also follow this combination with the vasovagal points or the autonomic heart points to cause a vasovagal faint or cardiac arrest.

Severe pain in the stomach can cause nausea, vomiting, and a vasovagal faint. When the radial nerve is attacked in combination with the opposite leg nerves, aberrant reference will cause the pain to be felt in the stomach. Thus, combining points on the radial nerve with points on the opposite leg nerves can cause nausea, vomiting, and a vasovagal faint. If a vasovagal point followed this combination, there would be a greater likelihood of causing a vasovagal faint or cardiac arrest because of summation. Aberrant reference combinations and the vasovagal points are synergistic because they both increase the parasympathetic effects on the heart. Additionally, if this combination were followed by an attack to a point connected to the same spinal level, the effect would be even greater because of facilitation. In this example, the points connected to the same spinal level include Bladder 16–19, Liver 14, Gall Bladder 24, and Spleen 21.

Stimulating the radial nerve through the large intestine, lung, and triple warmer points will set up the first four intercostal nerves and the first four dorsal nerve roots to affect the lung because of convergence. An attack to the points on the first four intercostal nerves either in combination with, or following, the points on the radial nerve will cause pain in the lungs as a result of stimulating the lung sympathetic nerves. This could lead to a vasovagal faint or a spasm of the intercostal muscles causing difficulty breathing. If this combination were followed by an attack to Large Intestine 17, the effects would be more likely to include a vasovagal faint or cardiac arrest because of convergence and facilitation. Attacking the Large Intestine 17 point stimulates the phrenic nerve, which is connected to the radial nerve by convergence at the C5 level of the spinal cord. When this nerve is attacked after the radial nerve, the effect is synergistic because the C5 level of the spinal cord will have been facilitated by the radial nerve attack. Additionally, because this combination can cause a vasovagal faint, a subsequent attack to the parasympathetic heart points would have synergistic effects. This example illustrates how multiple methods of increasing the parasympathetic effects on the heart are synergistic because of summation.

A simultaneous attack to the radial nerve, the phrenic nerve, and one of the first four intercostal nerves will most likely cause a vasovagal faint. There are two reasons for this effect. First, attacking these points can cause severe pain that indirectly stimulates nucleus tractus solitarii, leading to a vasovagal faint. Second, since all of these nerves can affect the lungs, they will cause an aberrant reference effect at the T1–4 level, which can stimulate the lung sympathetic nerves, resulting in severe pain. This will also stimulate the nucleus tractus solitarii, leading to a vasovagal faint. This illustrates an important concept: multiple methods of stimulating the nucleus tractus solitarii are synergistic when used together.

There are many other aspects of dim-mak that can be explained by medical science. Many have heard that the martial arts teach an individual to use an opponent's strength against him or her. Various styles teach that the secret to using this principle involves the use of body mechanics. However, an understanding of the neuroscience involved in dim-mak can explain how the martial artist can use the dim-mak points to exploit this principle. There are many different reflexes that occur in response to pain. For example, the body will always try to move the affected nerve away from the stimulus causing pain. This is called the withdrawal reflex. Pressing, grabbing, or striking a point usually causes pain. Thus, any time a point is attacked, the body will move in a direction opposite the angle of attack. If the opponent attempted to move toward the angle of attack, the stimulation of the nerve would increase. At a certain level of stimulation, the nerve would become very painful and the opponent's withdrawal reflex would cause him to move away. These reflexes redefine the use of this principle and are very effective when grappling.

The application of medical science to dim-mak also provides an explanation of how one can decrease an opponent's strength or cause paralysis. When a nerve is compressed or struck, the muscle that it controls will lose strength. This is called reflex paralysis. The point that controls a specific muscle is usually on a nerve that is in the area of the muscle but closer to the body. The use of reflex paralysis enables one to dislocate almost any joint as well as release any hold. Attacking the points on the radial nerve will cause an opponent to release his or her grip. If the Pericardium 2 point were attacked, the biceps would lose strength, making the elbow vulnerable to hyperextension. Consequently, the elbow joint could be easily hyperextended and dislocated as a result of pressure on the back of the elbow. The points on the wrist and forearm will weaken the wrist joint, leaving it vulnerable to dislocation. The points above the knee on the front and side of the leg will release the knee joint and allow it to be dislocated. Finally, the points on the upper back, armpit, and chest will enable the shoulder to be dislocated.

This chapter provided a basic overview of the medical science behind dim-mak. Mastering the medical concepts in this book will provide the reader with a strong foundation for studying the relationship between dim-mak and medical science. This can be an invaluable tool when attempting to find the dim-mak applications contained within the traditional forms. It can also help one to understand the effects of dim-mak on the body, which is conducive to grouping the points according to their effects on the nervous and cardiovascular systems. This simplifies the building of synergistic combinations and can be used to develop guidelines for combining points.

Chapter 9

Putting It All Together
Advanced

There is a great deal to be learned in studying the relationship between dim-mak and medical science. As with all aspects of the martial arts, this is a lifelong endeavor. Since attacking the heart is the most lethal aspect of dim-mak and because the purpose of this book is to illustrate the dangers inherent in dim-mak, this chapter will discuss advanced combinations affecting the heart. This includes advanced combinations without the arm points. Additionally, a few basic moves common to many styles will be discussed to illustrate the effectiveness of applying medical science to the study of dim-mak. It is not important to learn the specific combinations. One should focus on understanding how the medical concepts are applied.

A discussion of the advanced methods of applying the principles in this book to the study of dim-mak begins with the heart points on the arm. This includes the points on both the heart and pericardial meridians. These points will set up points on the head, neck, and body to affect the heart. The sympathetic stimulation of the heart is enhanced when an attack to these points is followed by an attack to the sympathetic heart points. Such a combination of points could easily induce ventricular fibrillation or a heart attack, both of which can be fatal. When the sympathetic heart points are followed by an attack to the autonomic heart points, there is an even greater probability of causing death.

The points on the ulnar and median nerves increase the sympathetic stimulation of the heart because they are connected to the cardiac sympathetic nerves by convergence. The sympathetic heart points on the chest and back have the same mechanism of action. This means that they are synergistic with the heart points on the arm. When attacked, the autonomic heart points can cause direct trauma to the heart, which, in the presence of increased sympathetic stimulation, can lead to ventricular fibrillation. In addition, increased sympathetic stimulation of the heart can cause a spasm of the coronary arteries resulting in a heart attack. As the level of sympathetic stimulation of the heart is increased, the probability of causing a lethal spasm of the coronary arteries also increases. Thus, when multiple heart points are used to increase the sympathetic stimulation of the heart, there is a greater probability of causing a heart attack or ventricular fibrillation.

The heart points on the arm can be followed by an attack to the parasympathetic heart points on the head and neck to cause a vasovagal faint or cardiac arrest. This combination is more effective than attacking the parasympathetic heart points alone and results in a greater probability of causing cardiac arrest. If this attack was ineffective or if one wanted to cause even greater damage, there are basically two choices: attack additional parasympathetic heart points for a synergistic parasympathetic effect or attack the autonomic heart points to cause heart block. The autonomic heart points could even be attacked after the additional parasympathetic heart points for an even greater effect. As more points are added, the probability of cardiac arrest increases proportionately.

In this example, the points on the ulnar and median nerves increase the sympathetic stimulation of the heart, which potentiates the parasympathetic points on the head and neck. The additional parasympathetic heart points work synergistically because of summation. The autonomic heart points have a greater likelihood of causing cardiac arrest because there is a greater probability of heart trauma causing cardiac arrest in the presence of increased parasympathetic activity.

The celiac plexus located under the Conception Vessel 14 point is an especially effective point for increasing parasympathetic effects on the heart. It is neurologically connected to all of the internal organs except the lungs and colon. Thus, it is synergistic with aberrant reference combinations that affect all but these two organs. This point can also affect the heart because it is connected to the T5 level of the spinal cord, which is directly connected to the cardiac sympathetic nerves. Additionally, because the celiac plexus increases the parasympathetic effects on the heart, it can be used as a vasovagal point. This means that it is potentiated by increased sympathetic stimulation of the heart and synergistic with any direct parasympathetic heart point. Thus, this point can be used with any point or combination that increases the parasympathetic effects on the heart. This includes aberrant reference combinations and the parasympathetic heart points.

The heart and pericardial points on the arm can also be used in combination with points on the body or legs to cause an aberrant reference effect on one of the internal organs. One has to understand the main combinations in order to effect a precise follow-up to a specific organ. However, certain general rules apply that make it very easy to affect the heart. When the heart or pericardial points are stimulated, they sensitize the heart sympathetic nerves because of convergence and facilitation. Attacking these points in combination with any of the body points above the last two ribs will have an aberrant reference effect on the heart. This includes the Bladder 11–20 points on the back as well as the points on the chest and upper abdomen. An aberrant reference combination affecting the heart can lead to a heart attack or cardiac arrest.

Since an aberrant reference combination increases the parasympathetic effects on the heart, it is synergistic with any other point that increases the parasympathetic effects on the heart. This includes points on the cranial nerves, the occipital nerves, the carotid sinus, and the celiac plexus. These points in any combination will magnify the parasympathetic effects on the heart and increase the probability of causing cardiac arrest. Additionally, because it increases the parasympathetic effects on the heart, an aberrant reference combination could be used to set up the autonomic heart points to cause heart block or cardiac arrest. The effect of an aberrant reference combination on the parasympathetic nervous system also explains why such an attack is potentiated by increased sympathetic stimulation of the heart.

Clearly there are many different methods of combining the heart points in a synergistic manner. The subject of combinations raises the issue of how many points should be attacked. When dealing with the heart, an attack to a single point could be fatal to a susceptible individual if it were hard enough. Attacking five points in what is known in Chinese medicine as the cycle of destruction has been postulated to have lethal effects. This is interesting, because one must attack at least five different points in order to apply all the principles of synergy based on Western medical science. When the heart is attacked with such a combination, death is an almost inevitable consequence. The following five steps illustrate the application of this concept:

- *Heart point on the arm*: An attack to one of the heart points on the arm will apply the concept of convergence and facilitate the cardiac sympathetic nerves. This alone could cause a heart attack in a susceptible individual.
- *Sympathetic heart point*: This point is synergistic with the first because they both increase the sympathetic stimula-

tion of the heart. Adding this point increases the likelihood of a heart attack and illustrates the principle of summation.

- *Parasympathetic heart point*: This point will be synergistic with the second because increased sympathetic stimulation of the heart potentiates the parasympathetic effects on the heart. Adding this point could result in cardiac arrest.

- *Parasympathetic heart point*: Adding a second parasympathetic heart point will be synergistic with the third point because of summation. Because the parasympathetic heart points are synergistic, adding this point further increases the likelihood of cardiac arrest.

- *Autonomic heart point*: Attacking one of the autonomic heart points when there are increased parasympathetic effects on the heart can cause cardiac arrest. Attacking two sympathetic heart points followed by two parasympathetic heart points will cause an extreme increase in the parasympathetic effects on the heart. Thus, when the autonomic heart point is attacked, the probability of cardiac arrest is further increased.

These five points will combine the concepts of convergence, summation, and facilitation with the magnification of the parasympathetic effects due to sympathetic stimulation and the increased likelihood that the autonomic heart points will cause cardiac arrest in the event of increased parasympathetic effects. In order for such a combination of points to be effective, these points must be attacked either simultaneously or in rapid succession. Points that have similar effects could be attacked together and followed by the next point. For example, the first and second points could be combined and followed by a combination of the third and fourth points. The fifth and final point should be attacked after the other four. In addition, the third or fourth point could be replaced with an aberrant reference combination, which will have similar effects on the heart.

This is probably the most lethal method of combining the dim-mak points. No one should ever have a need to take a confrontation to this extreme. This method of combining points has only been mentioned to illustrate the true danger of dim-mak and demonstrate how its effects can be substantiated by modern medical science. However, this method is certainly no secret, since there are movements in the traditional forms that can be used to attack the same combination of points. These combinations may or may not have been the original interpretation of the form's creator. Some of the combinations derived from forms follow both the cycle of destruction and the principles outlined in this book. Thus, it is conceivable that these techniques were created based on the five-element theory. It is interesting that one can find the same interpretation of a form by using both the five-element theory and medical science. Although there's no way to know for sure, this provides some evidence that the combinations derived from medical science could be the original interpretation of the traditional forms.

HEART ATTACK AND CARDIAC ARREST

All of the heart points have the potential to cause a heart attack, especially the sympathetic heart points. Not everyone who is attacked on the heart points will suffer a heart attack (i.e., a decrease in blood flow through a coronary artery leading to a state of cardiac oxygen deprivation, which results in the death of cardiac tissue), but it is always a possibility. This is especially true in men over 40. When the heart points are combined with a knockout technique, the probability of a heart attack increases dramatically. Medical science has found that increased sympathetic stimulation can cause a spasm of the coronary arteries.[1] This can cause a heart attack by itself. However, when this is combined with an attack to any point or combination that can cause a vasovagal faint, it is much more likely to cause a heart attack because the sudden drop in blood pressure will further decrease the blood flow to the heart. In such a situation, a heart attack is almost inevitable.

Cardiac arrest (i.e., cessation of the heartbeat) has also been mentioned many times, especially with any point or combination that increases the parasympathetic effects on the heart. In a susceptible individual, attacking any point that increases the parasympathetic effects can cause cardiac arrest. However, in most people cardiac arrest can only be induced with a drastic increase in the parasympathetic effects on the heart. This could be accomplished by setting up the parasympathetic heart points with the sympathetic heart points and by combining the parasympathetic heart points with each other or an aberrant reference combination.

DIM-MAK WITHOUT THE ARM POINTS

All of the methods of dim-mak mentioned so far have involved attacking the arm points. However, there are advanced methods of attacking the points that do not require the use of the arm points. The effectiveness of these methods is also substantiated by medical science. The easiest method of attacking an individual without using the arm points is to attack the vasovagal points on the head and neck in combination. Any one of these points can cause a vasovagal faint by itself, but this requires a great deal of force. There are two methods of getting around this. The first involves striking the same point multiple times. The second involves attacking multiple points. Multiple vasovagal points in combination are more likely to cause excessive stimulation of the nucleus tractus solitarii, leading to a vasovagal faint. As more vasovagal points are added to a combination, there is also an increased probability of causing cardiac arrest.

The same principles of setting up the parasympathetic effects on the heart with increased sympathetic stimulation can apply to vasovagal point combinations without the arm points. One could increase the sympathetic stimulation of the heart by attacking the sympathetic heart points on the body. Following this with an attack to multiple vasovagal points will most likely cause a vasovagal faint and possibly cardiac arrest. If one attacked the autonomic heart points after this combination, there would be an even greater chance of causing cardiac arrest.

The sympathetic heart points can also be followed by an attack to the autonomic heart points to induce ventricular fibrillation. However, most of the points on the chest connect to the T1–4 levels of the spinal cord, which also connect to the sympathetic nerves of the lung. The effect of striking the chest points that are on the nerves connected to these spinal levels without striking the arm points would be minimal because the sympathetic nerves would not be facilitated. There are two methods of getting around this dilemma. The first involves attacking the two sympathetic heart points on the neck: Small Intestine 17 and Large Intestine 17. These two points are located adjacent to sympathetic ganglions that connect directly to the heart and will cause a direct increase in the sympathetic stimulation of the heart as well as facilitation of the cardiac sympathetic nerves. This will cause the chest points to affect the heart when attacked.

The second method involves the points connected to the T5 level of the spinal cord, which include Stomach 18, Kidney 22, and Bladder 15. T5 is only connected to the cardiac sympathetic nerves, and attacking these points will directly increase the sympathetic effects on the heart. An attack to these points will also cause facilitation of the T5 level and the cardiac sympathetic nerves, which means it can cause an arrhythmia or heart attack. These effects will be increased when there is a prior increase in the sympathetic stimulation of the heart. As more points that increase the sympathetic stimulation of the heart are attacked, there is an increased probability of causing a heart attack. In addition, since these points increase the sympathetic stimulation of the heart and facilitate the cardiac sympathetic nerves, they will set up the other chest points to affect the heart when attacked. Thus, it is possible to set up and attack the heart with just the chest points. Once the sympathetic stimulation of the heart is increased, one could attack the autonomic heart points to cause ventricular fibrillation. Once again, as points are added with synergistic effects, the probability of causing death increases.

There is an advanced method of using the concept of aberrant reference to cause a vasovagal faint and possibly cardiac arrest. This method can be set up by any method that increases the sympathetic stimulation of the heart and potentiated by a follow-up attack to the parasympathetic heart points, the autonomic heart points, or both. As more points are added—either sympathetic points before or parasympathetic points after—the probability of causing cardiac arrest increases. Because one need not attack the arm points to use this method of aberrant reference, it enables the martial artist to launch a preemptive attack before the opponent strikes or grabs.

Attacking the Heart

Simultaneously striking the same point on both sides of the body: Stomach 17–18, Pericardium 1, Gall Bladder 22–23, Spleen 17, and Kidney 22–23. Because one is attacking the same point on both sides, the pain meets in the middle at the heart.

Simultaneously striking points diagonally: Heart 1, Lung 1, Gall Bladder 22–24, Spleen 17, or Pericardium 1 in combination diagonally with Liver 14, Spleen 21, or Stomach 17–18.

Simultaneously striking anterior and posterior points diagonally:

- Bladder 11-13 in combination with Liver 14, Gall Bladder 24, Stomach 17–18, or Conception Vessel 14.
- Bladder 14 in combination with Stomach 16–18, Conception Vessel 14, or Liver 14.
- Bladder 15 in combination with Stomach 16–18 or Conception Vessel 14.
- Bladder 13–15 in combination with Kidney 22–23 or Conception Vessel 17.

Attacking the Lungs

Simultaneously striking the same point on both sides of the body: Stomach 15–16 or Lung 1–2.

Attacking the Digestive System

Striking the same point on both sides of the body: Liver 14, Gall Bladder 24, or Spleen 21.

Simultaneously striking points diagonally:

- Stomach 16 or Kidney 24 in combination diagonally with Spleen 6 and 9–12; Gall Bladder 25, 31, and 41; Stomach 34, 36, 38, and 41; or liver 3, 6, and 11–13.
- Pericardium 1, Gall Bladder 22–23, or Stomach 17 in combination diagonally with Spleen 6 and 9–12, Gall Bladder 25 and 31, Stomach 34, or liver 6 and 11–13.
- Stomach 18, Spleen 17, or Kidney 22 in combination diagonally with Spleen 10–12, Gall Bladder 25 and 31, or Liver 12–13.
- Liver 14 in combination diagonally with Spleen 11–12, Gall Bladder 25, or Liver 12–13.
- Gall Bladder 24 or Spleen 21 in combination diagonally with Spleen 12, Gall Bladder 25, or Liver 12–13.

Simultaneously striking anterior and posterior points diagonally:

(Since these points involve the dorsal nerve roots, the lung and heart can both be affected.)

- Bladder 13 in combination with Spleen 6 and 9–12; Gall Bladder 25, 31, and 41; Stomach 34, 36, 38, and 41; Kidney 6 and 8, or Liver 3, 6, and 11–13.
- Bladder 14 in combination with Spleen 6 and 9–12; Gall Bladder 25 and 31; Stomach 34; Kidney 6 and 8, or Liver 6 and 11–13.
- Bladder 15 in combination front to back diagonally with Spleen 10–12, Gall Bladder 25 and 31, or Liver 12–13.
- Bladder 16 in combination front to back diagonally with Spleen 11–12, Gall Bladder 25, or Liver 12–13.
- Bladder 17 in combination front to back diagonally with Spleen 12, Gall Bladder 25, or Liver 12–13.

BASIC MOVEMENTS TURNED DEADLY

The final aspect of applying medical science to the study of dim-mak involves the application of dim-mak and medical science to the traditional forms. Thus, some techniques that are common to many styles will be analyzed for dim-mak applications that can be explained by modern medical science.

There are many styles that have some form of middle block followed by a punch. Some styles use a closed fist with linear movements and others use open hands with circular movements. This combination of a middle block and punch can be a very effective method of attacking the dim-mak points. The following explanation assumes that one is going to middle block with the right hand and punch with the left hand. The points used are illustrated in Photos A1 and A2.

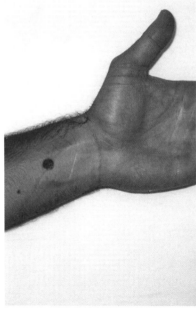
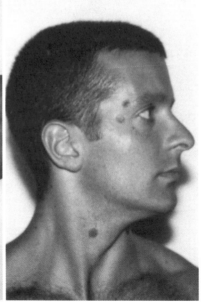

PHOTO A1: Pericardium 6.

PHOTO A2: Triple Warmer 23, Gall Bladder 1, and Stomach 9.

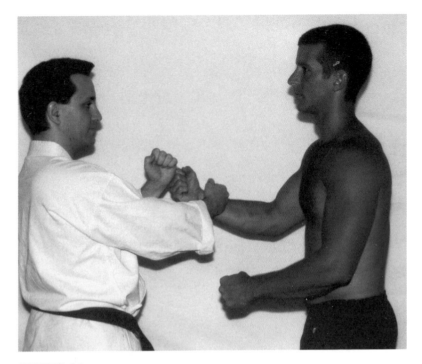

PHOTO A3

Movement 1: When the right hand crosses the body to the set position it can actually be attacking the Pericardium 6 point on the right hand of the attacker (see Photo A3). This will stimulate the median nerve, which will increase the sympathetic stimulation of the heart due to convergence.

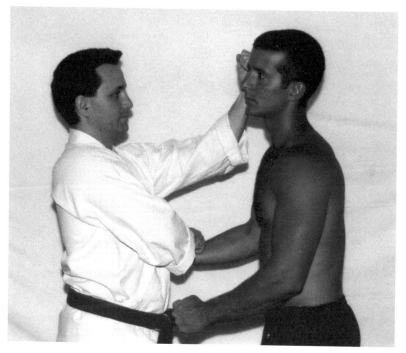

PHOTO A4

Movement 2: Just after movement 1, the left hand comes across and strikes the Triple Warmer 23 point from left to right and slightly forward (see Photo A4). This will stimulate one of the cranial nerves, which will increase the parasympathetic effects on the heart and could cause a vasovagal faint. This point is enhanced by the increased sympathetic stimulation from movement 1.

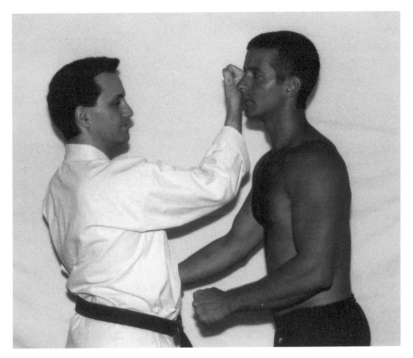

PHOTO A5

Movement 3: The right hand comes up and strikes the opponent's right eyeball with a backfist (see Photo A5). This will cause an oculocardiac reflex, which will also increase the parasympathetic effects on the heart. This could cause a vasovagal faint by itself. However, it is more effective after movements 1 and 2 because of the increased sympathetic stimulation of the heart from movement 1 and the synergistic effect with movement 2 due to summation. At this point, a vasovagal faint is very likely and cardiac arrest is a possibility. If the eyeball were ruptured, there would be irreversible blindness in the right eye.

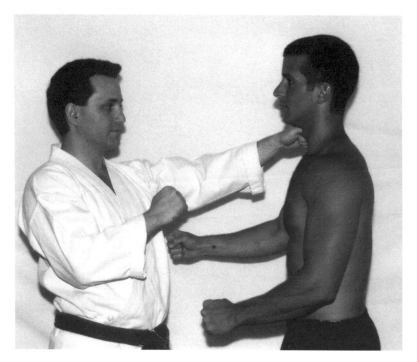

PHOTO A6

Movement 4: The left fist punches the opponent's right carotid sinus point with an extended foreknuckle (see Photo A6). This point will be synergistic because it further increases the parasympathetic effects on the heart. At this point, a vaso-vagal faint is most definite and cardiac arrest is very likely.

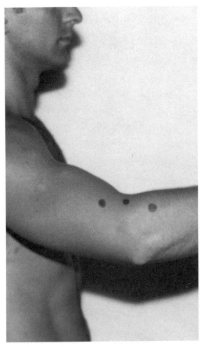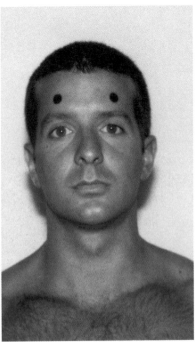

PHOTO B1: Large Intestine 10, 12, and 13.   **PHOTO B2: Gall Bladder 14.**

This example illustrates how a basic movement common to almost all styles can be very deadly and dangerous when the medical concepts of dim-mak are applied to its interpretation. The lethal effectiveness and danger of this technique also explains why it is common to so many forms. The creators of the forms probably wanted to include it in their katas because they knew this or an even deadlier interpretation.

There are many other examples of applying these concepts to the study of dim-mak and forms. One very common technique involves a palm strike to the Gall Bladder 14 point in combination with a strike to the arm points, as follows (points used are illustrated in Photos B1 and B2).

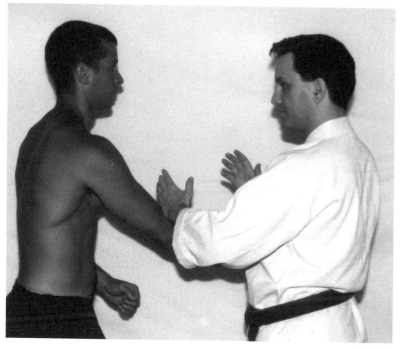

PHOTO B3

Movement 1: Attacker punches, pushes, or grabs with his right hand. The defender's left hand strikes one of the large intestine points on his opponent's right arm (see Photo B3). This attacks the radial nerve, causing pain, which increases the sympathetic stimulation of the heart through a somatosympathetic reflex.

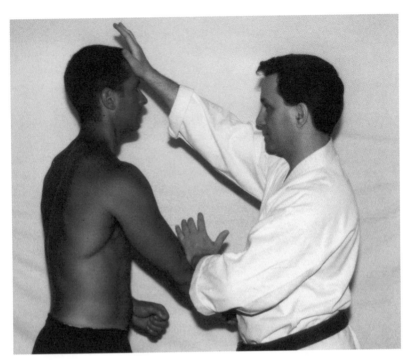

PHOTO B4

Movement 2: The right hand strikes the Gall Bladder 14 point (see Photo B4). This attacks the supraorbital nerve, which is one of the cranial nerves. This nerve can cause a vasovagal faint and increased parasympathetic stimulation of the heart by itself. However, when there is increased sympathetic stimulation of the heart, it is much more likely to cause a vasovagal faint and could cause cardiac arrest.

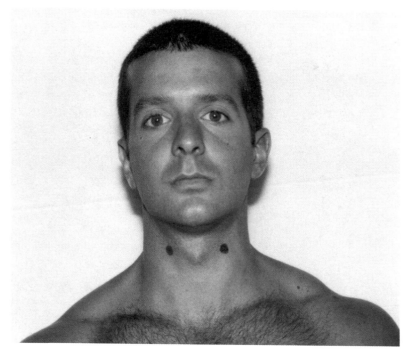

PHOTO C1: Stomach 9.

Another very common technique familiar to many styles involves a strike with the edge of the hand. This is usually referred to as a knife-edge or shuto strike. This technique can also be deadly when the principles of medical science are applied to its interpretation. Those who teach dim-mak use this technique to strike the opponent's attacking arm with one hand and the carotid sinus point with the other. In this example, the attacker is punching, pushing, or grabbing with the right hand. The points used are illustrated in Photos A1 (p. 137) and C1.

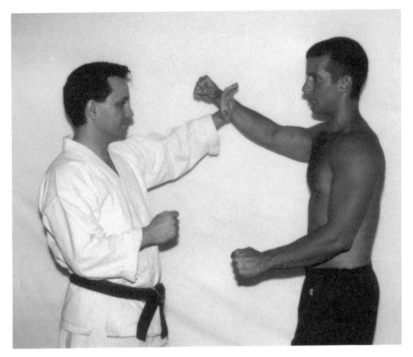

PHOTO C2

Movement 1: The left hand strikes the Pericardium 6 point with the edge of the hand (see Photo C2). This attacks the median nerve and increases the sympathetic stimulation of the heart through convergence and a somatosympathetic reflex.

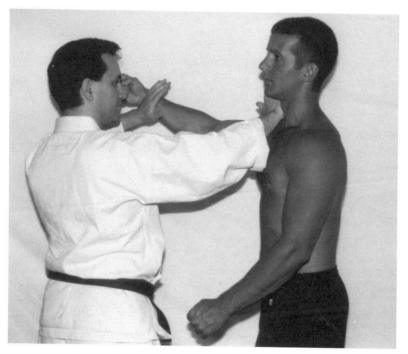

PHOTO C3

Movement 2: The edge of the right hand strikes the Stomach 9 point (see Photo C3). This attacks the carotid sinus, which can cause a vasovagal faint or cardiac arrest by itself. However, its effects are enhanced by the increased sympathetic stimulation of the heart caused by Movement 1.

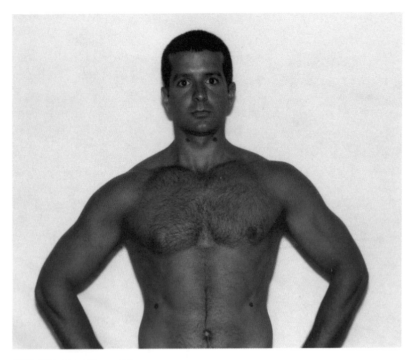

PHOTO C4: Liver 13.

There is another version of this technique in which one is taught a set position followed by a block with the edge of the hand. If one understands the concepts of convergence, aberrant reference, and summation, it becomes clear how this can be very deadly. In this example, the attacker is again punching, pushing, or grabbing with the right hand. The points used are illustrated in Photos A1 (p. 137), C1 (p. 145**)**, and C4.

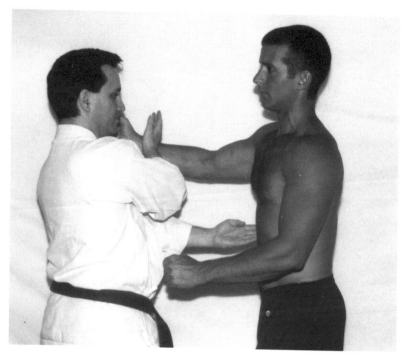

PHOTO C5

Movement 1: The edge of right hand strikes the Pericardium 6 point toward the defender (see Photo C5). This attacks the median nerve and causes an increase in the sympathetic stimulation of the heart and facilitation of the cardiac sympathetic nerves. This registers at the T1 level of the spinal cord.

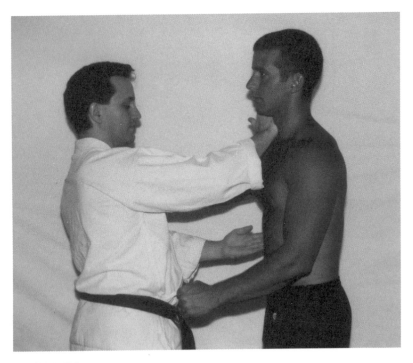

PHOTO C6

Movement 2: The fingers of the left hand stab into the
Liver 13 point (see Photo C5). (This movement is simultaneous with Movement 1.) Attacking the Liver 13 point stimulates the tenth intercostal nerve, which causes pain at the T10
level of the spinal cord. When this nerve is attacked simultaneously with the median nerve, aberrant reference causes the
pain to be displaced to the T5 level of the spinal cord. This
can result in the brain's interpreting the pain as coming from
the heart, which can cause a vasovagal faint or cardiac arrest.

Movement 3: The edge of the right hand strikes the
Stomach 9 point (see Photo C6). This attacks the carotid
sinus, which will be much more likely to cause cardiac arrest
in addition to a vasovagal faint because of the increased
parasympathetic effects from the aberrant reference effect of
Movements 1 and 2.

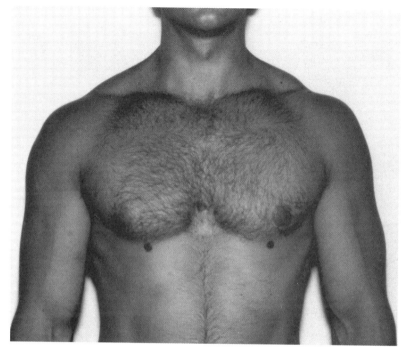

PHOTO D1: Stomach 18.

Many forms contain a series of three punches. If these punches were used to attack the heart points on the chest, they could be lethal. In this example, the defender grabs his opponent's right arm at the wrist with the first punch. This could be the result of parrying an attack or just a grab. The points used are illustrated in Photos A1 (p. 137) and D1.

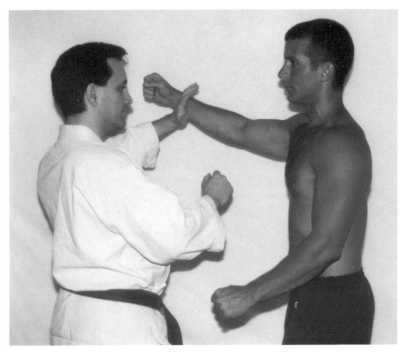

PHOTO D2

Movement 1: The left hand strikes the opponent's Pericardium 6 point (see Photo D2) and then grabs the opponent's left wrist and grinds Heart 7 point into the bone and pulls it. This action stimulates the median and ulnar nerves. This increases the sympathetic stimulation of the heart and facilitates the cardiac sympathetic nerves.

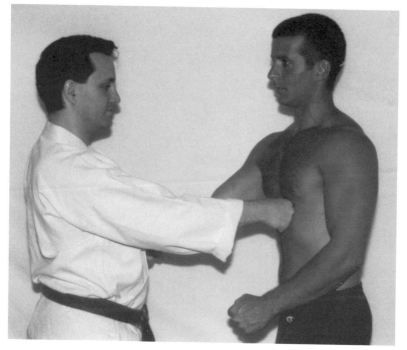

PHOTO D3

Movement 2: With a single knuckle, the right hand punches the Stomach 18 point on the left side of the opponent (see Photo D3). This attacks the fifth intercostal nerve, which is connected to cardiac sympathetic nerves at the T5 level of the spinal cord. The Stomach 18 point has the same effects as the Heart 7 point. The combination of these two points results in a greater increase in the sympathetic stimulation of the heart because of summation. This could result in a heart attack or ventricular fibrillation.

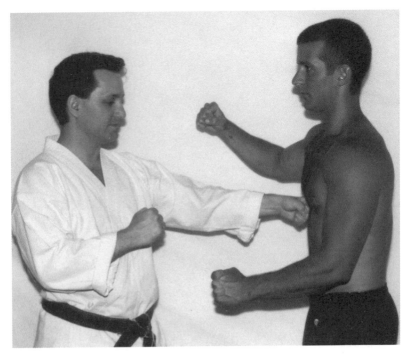

PHOTO D4

Movement 3: With a single knuckle, the left hand punch-es the Stomach 18 point on the right side of the opponent (see Photo D4). This attacks the fifth intercostal nerve on the opposite side of the body. This point has the same effects as the previous two points and results in an even greater increase in the sympathetic stimulation of the heart because the T5 level was facilitated by attacking the first two points. This exaggerated increase in the sympathetic stimulation of the heart is more likely to cause ventricular fibrillation or a heart attack.

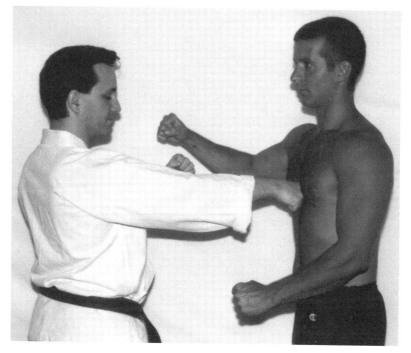

PHOTO D5

Movement 4: With a single knuckle, the right hand punches the Kidney 22 point (see Photo D5). This is an autonomic heart point, which has been set up to cause ventricular fibrillation and death by the increased sympathetic stimulation of the heart. This point can also further increase the sympathetic stimulation of the heart, which could cause a heart attack.

There are numerous combinations and methods of attack. This text is not intended to be a listing of all the possible methods of attacking the dim-mak points. Rather it is intended to be a guide that will assist the reader in understanding the effects of a dim-mak technique based on modern medicine. The combinations of points discussed are intended to illustrate the medical concepts behind dim-mak. The ancient masters handed down a precious gift to modern martial artists by passing on their methods of attacking the points in their forms. These methods were based on battle experience in combination with acupuncture theories. The medical science behind dim-mak will enable the modern martial artist to discover the secrets of dim-mak that are contained within these forms. Although it is true that one can never really be sure of the original meaning of a form, the study of medical science and dim-mak will enable the modern martial artist to develop very effective dim-mak interpretations. Furthermore, an understanding of the medical science behind dim-mak will enable the martial artist to determine how effective an application is without dangerous experimentation on others.

Chapter 10

Revival and Healing

The martial arts have always been influenced by the concept of yin and yang. Nowhere is this more evident than in the healing aspects of dim-mak. Learning revival is as much a part of dim-mak as yin is a part of yang. Perhaps this is the reason that healing has always been a part of the martial arts. The truly balanced and humane martial artist should know how to reverse whatever damage he is capable of causing. In dim-mak, there are acupuncture-based revival methods for organ dysfunction, cardiac arrest, pain, and loss of consciousness. Although these methods are far from flawless, their existence says a great deal about the true nature of the martial arts. Therefore, this chapter will examine the ancient revival methods from the perspective of medical science.

Massage and acupuncture are the most common methods of healing the damage inflicted by dim-mak. These methods have been proven to be effective through years of practice, and there is a neurological basis for their efficacy. Massage and acupuncture can actually reverse dim-mak's effects on the autonomic nervous system by blocking nerve signals in the spinal cord. There are two types of nerve fibers that sense pain: type A and type C. Stimulating a point with a needle or massage activates only the type A nerve fibers because they have a low threshold. Conversely, when a point is attacked, the type C nerve fibers are activated because they have a high threshold. Medical research has found that stimulation of the type A nerves can block the pain signal from the type C nerves in the spinal cord. Using acupuncture or massage on a point stimulates the type A nerve fibers, which then block the effects of a dim-mak attack by interrupting the pain signal from the type C nerves. This phenomenon is known in neurology as central inhibition of pain due to counter irritation. (See Figure 21.)

Some revival methods use the sympathetic nervous system to reverse the damage of dim-mak. The effects of the sym-

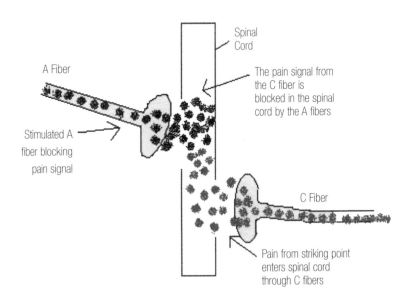

FIGURE 21
Central inhibition of pain due to counter irritation.

pathetic nervous system are mainly due to chemicals called epinephrine and norepinephrine, which are neurotransmitters. There are revival methods that purposely inflict pain by pressing or pinching the points on the ends of the fingers and toes to arouse a lethargic person. This results in a somatosympathetic reflex, which increases the blood levels of epinephrine and norepinephrine. These neurotransmitters then cause an increase in blood pressure and stimulation of the central nervous system. As a result, the person feels much more awake and alert.

To reverse the effects of a vasovagal faint, the Gall Bladder 20 points are pressed. There are reports in the medical literature of neuralgia (pain) in the occipital nerves causing autonomic failure.[1] This means that pain introduced into these nerves can slow or stop the activity of the autonomic nervous system. Thus, if one caused a vasovagal faint from excessive parasympathetic activity, stimulating the lesser occipital nerve through the Gall Bladder 20 point could inhibit this activity and allow the body to stabilize.

Another method of reviving a vasovagal faint involves slapping the trapezium muscle on the back of the neck. This stimulates the spinal accessory nerve and will arouse an unconscious person because the spinal accessory nerve has branches that are connected to the ascending reticular activating system. Stimulation of this area of the brain is the main mechanism that the body uses to arouse an individual from sleep. Thus, slapping the spinal accessory nerve stimulates the reticular activating system, thereby arousing the person from a loss of consciousness. Furthermore, the spinal accessory nerve is neurologically connected to the occipital nerves. Slapping the spinal accessory nerve could have an effect on the occipital nerves in addition to the reticular activating system. Conversely, stimulating the occipital nerves could have an effect on the reticular activating system. Because of this, these two methods are synergistic when used together.

There is a method of reversing a dim-mak-induced cardiac

arrest, but it has not been scientifically proven to be as effective as CPR. The question of which method is the most effective for a dim-mak-induced cardiac arrest shall remain unanswered for the present time. The ancient method will only be discussed for the sake of education. This in no way implies that the author endorses its use.

The technique involves an open hand slap to the right side of the back between the spine and the scapula at the levels of the 3rd, 4th, and 5th thoracic vertebrae. This area corresponds to the bladder 13, 14, and 15 points and will directly stimulate the sympathetic nerves connected to the heart. This will cause a release of epinephrine and norepinephrine directly into the heart, resulting in an increase in blood pressure, heart rate, and contractility. It is conceivable that this method could restart the heart after cardiac arrest. In fact, the advanced cardiac life-support protocol for cardiac arrest calls for an injection of epinephrine and CPR.

One should only strike the bladder points on the right side of the back because those on the left side can cause an arrhythmia. In addition, if the strike were too hard, it could result in cardiac arrest, an arrhythmia, or a heart attack. The best method involves using a blunt slap with the palm to avoid overstimulating the nerves. This technique could also be used to reverse the decrease in blood pressure and heart rate caused by a vasovagal faint technique because it directly reverses the parasympathetic effects on the heart. However, one should never strike these points immediately after attacking any points that affect the heart because this could lead to a heart attack or cardiac arrest.

When dealing with the revival of the heart, it is important to address the effects of the autonomic heart points. These points can cause commotio cordis, which has an extremely poor prognosis. Most victims of commotio cordis die even with CPR.[2,3] The few documented cases of survival all involved immediate CPR by trained professionals with either electronic defibrillation or a pericardial thump.[4,5] In this setting, the ancient revival methods are unproven and CPR has limited efficacy. Thus, one should avoid the misconception that dim-mak's effects are always reversible.

As evidenced by the revival of the heart, the sympathetic nervous system can actually reverse the effects of the parasympathetic nervous system. Interestingly, the reverse is also true. The parasympathetic nervous system can reverse the effects of the sympathetic nervous system. One can massage the carotid sinus to prevent an arrhythmia from occurring, or to stop certain forms of arrhythmias. Physicians routinely use many techniques to stimulate the parasympathetic effects on the heart in order to stop arrhythmias. They are called vagal maneuvers, and the most popular is carotid massage. Research has shown that vagal stimulation will decrease the incidence of ventricular fibrillation and ventricular tachycardia in the presence of increased sympathetic stimulation of the heart.[6] However, this method is ineffective in treating ventricular fibrillation once it has already started. The appropriate treatment for ventricular fibrillation is electronic defibrillation in a hospital.

It has been shown that many techniques can cause stimulation of the sympathetic nerves connected to the internal organs, resulting in somatovisceral reflexes and decreased blood flow. One can decrease the sympathetic stimulation of the internal organs by manipulating the dorsal nerve roots under the bladder points (see fig. 10). This method involves firm, steady pressure with the fingers about one inch from the spine bilaterally on the bladder points corresponding to the stimulated organ. The pressure should be firm but not painful and held until one feels a softening under the fingers. This is known in modern medicine as paraspinal inhibition, and it has been shown to decrease the sympathetic stimulation of the internal organs and restore normal blood flow.

Although the ancient revival methods can be explained by modern medical science, their efficacy remains unproven. The revival method used to block pain seems to be a safe and effective treatment. This is also true concerning the treatment of a somatovisceral reflex. There is evidence that the revival methods for a vasovagal faint can interrupt the effects of the autonomic nervous system and stimulate the arousal center in the brain. These methods seem to be very effective at reviving someone from a "knockout." Even the revival of the heart seems to be effective when it is explained by modern medical science. However, there is no dim-mak revival method that has the proven efficacy of CPR and advanced cardiac life-support. Thus, one is faced with a dilemma when dealing with the revival of a dim-mak attack. Should one use the ancient methods or seek medical attention? In the event of cardiac arrest, ventricular fibrillation, or a heart attack, one should call for help, administer CPR if there is no pulse, and seek medical treatment as soon as possible. The modern medical treatments for the heart are more effective and have proven efficacy. As for the revival methods for pain and knockouts, they seem to be effective, but the issues of safety and efficacy remain unsettled. Perhaps the ideal treatment for any dim-mak attack is to see both a physician and an acupuncturist.

Epilogue

Because modern medicine can provide an alternative explanation for dim-mak's effects, the ancient explanations and teachings might seem to be of questionable value. This is certainly not the case, for the traditional teachings and katas contain a wealth of information derived from combat experience. Ideally, the martial artist would benefit from both the traditional teachings and modern medicine. This can be accomplished by using medical science to analyze the traditional katas. In addition, one could use medical science to find the most effective dim-mak applications of a particular movement without experimenting on anyone. If an application seemed ineffective, one could slightly alter the technique to make it more effective or search for a different application. Some might argue that this could change how the traditional techniques are applied. While this may be true, it is relatively insignificant because change has always been a part of the martial arts.

Throughout marital arts history there have been multiple changes attributed to different cultures.

The Chinese martial arts where modified when they were introduced into Okinawa, and then the Okinawan martial arts were modified when they were introduced into Japan. Furthermore, the ancient masters would make changes in their art based on personal experience. Thus, the history of the martial arts is really a story of change and development. Dim-mak was derived from ancient acupuncture theories, and its effects were originally attributed to disruptions in a person's internal energy. Modern medical science can provide an alternative explanation. If the ancient martial arts were based on ancient medicine, then perhaps the modern martial arts should be based on modern medicine.

In the martial arts, there is a concept of a student completing a circle as he progresses from a novice to an expert. It is not until the advanced level that one realizes how much more there is to the mastery of an art. The real study of the martial arts begins at this advanced level. When one has learned both the traditional aspects of dim-mak and the concepts of medical science relating to dim-mak, the true journey begins. The application of medical science to the study of dim-mak could enable the advanced martial artist to reach the highest level of mastery: the level at which he develops his own methods of attacking the points.

This concept is not as outrageous as it may seem. At some point in time, a person came up with the idea of striking the acupuncture points. There was also an individual who devised the first kata. These people were human beings and not any more capable than modern man. However, in order to be able to develop one's own methods of attacking the points, one must first master the traditional forms, the dim-mak applications, and the medical science relating to dim-mak. Mastery is not the ability to perform katas or fluency in the vocabulary of medical science. It is a deep understanding of the principles behind both, and it requires a lifetime of study. A good teacher can be an invaluable asset in this endeavor.

The martial arts have always been corrupted by a great

deal of dogma, which has hindered their progression. Many egos have been swelled by the authority to order a student to do something without questioning. The martial artist should be skeptical of this approach to instruction. Students should be encouraged to do their own research and question their teaching. The student armed with knowledge will be able to quickly identify the inept instructor. Any teacher who is threatened by questioning is probably lacking in knowledge as well as humility. A knowledgeable instructor who knows the true meaning of the martial arts will be unthreatened by a student seeking knowledge.

The application of medical science to the study of dim-mak can serve as a catalyst for change. In addition to improving dim-mak techniques and eliminating inept teachers, it can alter the manner in which the traditional forms are taught. As this text has illustrated, medical science can explain how dim-mak can cause a loss of consciousness, organ dysfunction, and death. However, certain aspects of dim-mak remain a mystery. There is an internal aspect of a dim-mak strike that cannot be described in a book. One has to experience the sensation of internal energy, also known as chi or ki, in order to understand it. Perhaps medical science will elucidate this area sometime in the future. However, if the ancient teachings were correct about the dangers of dim-mak, they may very well be correct about the more esoteric aspects of the martial arts. The question is whether or not it really matters. After all, the real benefit of the martial arts is not the ability to fight, but rather the perfection of one's character.

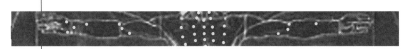

Endnotes

Introduction

1. McCarthy, *The Bible of Karate, Bubishi* (Rutland, Vt., and Tokyo: Charles E. Tuttle Company, Inc., 1995), 108–109.
2. McCarthy, *Bible*, 110–111, 129.
3. McCarthy, *Bible*, 26.
4. McCarthy, *Bible*, 107–147.
5. Owens and O'Brian, "Hypotension in Patients with Coronary Artery Disease: Can Profound Hypotension Cause Myocardial Ischemic Events?," Heart 82:4 (October 1999), 477.
6. DiGiovanna and Schiowitz, *An Osteopathic Approach to Diagnosis and Treatment* (Philadelphia: J.B. Lippincott, 1991), 2–3.

Chapter 1: Science or Science Fiction?

1. Samuels M.D., "Neurally Induced Cardiac Damage: Definition of the Problem," *Neurologic Clinics: Neurocardiology* 11:2 (May 1993) 284.
2. Link, Wang, Pandian, Bharati, Udelson, Lee, Vecchiotti, Mirra, Maron, and Estes III, "An Experimental Model of Sudden Death Due to Low Energy Chest Wall Impact (Commotio Cordis)," *New England Journal of Medicine* 338:25 (June 1998), 1809.
3. Natelson and Chang, "Sudden Death: A Neurocardiologic Phenomenon," *Neurologic Clinics: Neurocardiology* 11:2 (May 1993), 293.

Chapter 2: The Nervous System

1. Sato, "Neural Mechanisms of Autonomic Responses Elicited by Somatic Sensory Stimulation," *Neuroscience Behavior Physiology* 27:5, United States (Sept.–Oct. 1997), 610–621.
2. Sato, "Neural Mechanisms," 610–621.
3. DiGiovanna and Schiowitz, *An Osteopathic Approach to Diagnosis and Treatment* (Philadelphia: J.B. Lippincott, 1991), 15–16.

4. Samuels, "Neurally Induced Cardiac Damage: Definition of the Problem," *Neurologic Clinics: Neurocardiology* 11:2 (May 1993), 284.
5. Burns, "Visceral-Somatic and Somato-Visceral Spinal Reflexes," *The Journal of The American Osteopathic Association* 7:2 (October 1907), 54–55.
6. Waldman and Willie, *Interventional Pain Management* (Philadelphia: Saunders, 1996), 12.
7. Adams, Victor, and Ropper, *Principles of Neurology*, 6th ed., (New York: McGraw-Hill, 1997), 139.

Chapter 3: The Points
1. Morillo, Ellenbogen, and Fernando, "Pathophysiologic Basis for Vasodepressor Syncope," *Cardiology Clinics* 11:2 (May 1997), 233–249.
2. Talman and Kelkar, "Neural Control of the Heart: Central and Peripheral," *Neurologic Clinics: Neurocardiology* 11:2 (May 1992), 243.

Chapter 4: Methods of Attacking
1. Galer, "Painful Polyneuropathy." *Neurologic Clinics: Neurocardiology* 16:4 (Nov. 1998), 794.
2. Talman and Kelkar, "Neural Control of the Heart: Central and Peripheral," *Neurologic Clinics: Neurocardiology* 11:2 (May 1993), 243.

Chapter 5: A Medical Knockout
1. Diehl, Linden, and Chalkiadaki, "Cerebrovascular Mechanisms in Neurocardiogenic Syncope with and without Postural Tachycardia Syndrome," *Journal of the Autonomic Nervous System* 76:2 (1999), 159–166.
2. Morrillo, Ellenbogen, and Fernando, "Pathophysiologic Basis for Vasodepressor Syncope," *Cardiology Clinics* 11:2 (May 1997), 233–249.
3. Samuels, "Neurally Induced Cardiac Damage: Definition of the Problem," *Neurologic Clinics: Neurocardiology* 11:2 (May 1993), 275.
4. Samuels, "Neurally Induced," 275.
5. Gottesman, Ibrahim, Elfenbein, Mechanic, and Hertz, "Cardiac Arrest Caused by Trigeminal Neuralgia," *Headache* 36:6, United States (June 1996), 392–394.
6. Kuchta, Koulousakis, Decker, and Klug, "Pressor and Depressor Responses in Thermocoagulation of the Trigeminal Ganglion," *British Journal of Neurosurgery* 12:5, England (October 1995), 409–413.
7. Adams, Victor, and Ropper, *Principles of Neurology*, 6th ed., (New York: McGraw-Hill, 1997), 546.
8. Uryvaev, Iudel'son, and Sergeev, "Changes in Hemostasis and Vagal Tonus in Healthy Individuals and Patients with Facial Neuropathy by Micro-dose Heparin Stimulation of Nasal Receptors," *Vestin Ross Akad. Med. Nauk.* 8, Russia (1991), 22–23.
9. Bleasdale-Barr and Mathias, "Neck and Other Muscle Pains in Autonomic Failure: Their Association with Orthostatic Hypotension," *Journal of the Royal Society of Medicine* 91:7 (July 1998), 355–359.
10. Talman and Kelkar, "Neural Control of the Heart: Central and Peripheral," *Neurologic Clinics: Neurocardiology* 11:2 (May 1993), 243.

Chapter 6: Attacking the Internal Organs
1. Samuels, "Neurally Induced Cardiac Damage: Definition of the Problem,"

Neurologic Clinics: Neurocardiology 11:2 (May 1993), 284, 287.

2. Samuels, "Neurally Induced," 284, 287.

3. DiGiovanna and Schiowitz, *An Osteopathic Approach to Diagnosis and Treatment* (Philadelphia: J.B. Lippincott, 1991), 15–16.

4. Fauci et al, *Harrison's Principles of Internal Medicine*, 14th ed. (New York: McGraw-Hill, 1998), 217.

5. Samuels, "Neurally Induced Cardiac Damage: Definition of the Problem," *Neurologic Clinics: Neurocardiology* 11:2 (May 1993), 278.

6. Samuels, "Neurally Induced," 281.

7. Fauci, et al, *Harrison's Principles*, 217.

8. Fauci, et al, *Harrison's Principles*, 217.

9. Fauci, et al, *Harrison's Principles*, 217.

10. Kuchera and Kuchera, *Osteopathic Considerations in Systemic Dysfunction*, 2nd ed. (Columbus, Ohio: Greyden Press, 1994), 84.

11. Fauci, et al, *Harrison's Principles*, 2326.

12. Fauci, et al, *Harrison's Principles*, 2392.

13. Fauci, et al, *Harrison's Principles*, 1469.

14. Barker, Burton, and Zieve, *Principles of Ambulatory Medicine*, 5th ed. (Philadelphia: Williams and Wilkins, 1999), 642.

Chapter 7: The Heart

1. Kubertur and Franc, *Neurocardiology* (Mount Kisco, N.Y.: Futura Publishing Company, 1999), 125.

2. Fauci, et al, *Harrison's Principles*, 1374.

3. Fauci, et al, *Harrison's Principles*, 1352.

4. Robbins, Kumar, and Cotran, *Pathologic Basis of Disease*, 5th ed. (Philadelphia: Saunders, 1994) 530.

5. Fauci, et al, *Harrison's Principles*, 1352.

6. Sato, Sato, Suzuki., and Kimura. "A and C Reflexes Elicited in Cardiac Sympathetic Nerves by Single Shock to a Somatic Afferent Nerve Include Spinal and Supraspinal Components in Anesthetized Rats," *Neuroscience Research Journal* 25:1 (May 1996), 91–96.

7. Talman and Kelkar, "Neural Control of the Heart: Central and Peripheral," *Neurologic Clinics: Neurocardiology* 11:2 (May 1993), 248.

8. Kuchera and Kuchera, *Osteopathic Considerations in Systemic Dysfunction*, 2nd ed. (Columbus Ohio: Greyden Press, 1994), 57.

9. Kuchera and Kuchera, *Osteopathic Considerations*, 57.

10. Adams and Ropper, *Principles of Neurology*, 6th ed. (New York: McGraw-Hill, 1997), 546.

11. Natelson and Chang, "Sudden Death: A Neurocardiologic Phenomenon," *Neurologic Clinics: Neurocardiology* 11:2 (May 1993), 293.

12. Natelson and Chang, "Sudden Death," 294.

13. Talman and Kelkar, "Neural Control," 248.

14. Talman and Kelkar, "Neural Control," 243.

15. Maron, Link, Wang, and Estes, "Clinical Profile of Commotio Cordis: An Under Appreciated Cause of Sudden Death in the Young During Sports and Other Activities," *Journal of Cardiovascular Electrophysiology* 10:1, United States (July 1999), 114–120.

16. Denton and Kelelkar, "Homicidal Commotio Cordis in Two Children," *Journal of Forensic Science* 45:3, United States (May 2000), 734–735.
17. Maron, Poliac, Kaplan, and Mueller, "Blunt Impact to the Chest Leading to Sudden Death from Cardiac Arrest during Sports Activities," *New England Journal of Medicine* 333:6 (August 1995), 337–340.
18. Maron, Link, Wang, and Estes, "Clinical Profile," 120.
19. Maron, Poliac, Kaplan, and Mueller, "Blunt Impact," 339–340.
20. Link, Wang, Pandian, Bharati, Udelson, Lee, Vecchiotti, Mirra, Maron, and Estes, "An Experimental Model of Sudden Death Due to Low Energy Chest Wall Impact (Commotio Cordis)," *New England Journal of Medicine* 338: 25 (June 1998), 1809.
21. Link, Wang, Pandian, Bharati, Udelson, Lee, Vecchiotti, Mirra, Maron, and Estes, "An Experimental Model," 1809.
22. Link, Wang, Pandian, Bharati, Udelson, Lee, Vecchiotti, Mirra, Maron, and Estes, "An Experimental Model, 1809.
23. Link, Wang, Pandian, Bharati, Udelson, Lee, Vecchiotti, Mirra, Maron, and Estes, "An Experimental Model, 1809.
24. Maron, Link, Wang, and Estes, "Clinical Profile," 118, 120.
25. Link, Wang, Pandian, Bharati, Udelson, Lee, Vecchiotti, Mirra, Maron, and Estes, "An Experimental Model," 1806.
26. Link, Wang, Pandian, Bharati, Udelson, Lee, Vecchiotti, Mirra, Maron, and Estes, "An Experimental Model," 1806–1807.
27. Talman and Kelkar, "Neural Control," 243.

Chapter 9: Putting It All Together: Advanced

1. Michael L. Kuchera D.O. and William A. Kuchera D.O., *Osteopathic Considerations in Systemic Dysfunction*, 2nd ed. (Columbus, Ohio: Greyden Press, 1994), 55.

Chapter 10: Revival and Healing

1. Bleasdale-Barr and Mathias, "Neck and Other Muscle Pains in Autonomic Failure: Their Association with Orthostatic Hypotension," *Journal of the Royal Society of Medicine* 91:7 (July 1998): 355–359.
2. Maron, Poliac, Kaplan, and Mueller, "Blunt Impact to the Chest Leading to Sudden Death from Cardiac Arrest during Sports Activities," *New England Journal of Medicine* 333:6 (August 1995), 339.
3. Maron, Link, Wang, and Estes, "Clinical Profile of Commotio Cordis: An Under Appreciated Cause of Sudden Death in the Young during Sports and Other Activities," *Journal of Cardiovascular Electrophysiology* 10:1, United States (July 1999m), 118.
4. Link, Ginsburg, Wang, Kirchhoffer, Berul, Estes, and Paris, "Commotio Cordis: Cardiovascular Manifestations of a Rare Survivor," *Chest* 114: 1 (July 1998), 326–328.
5. Maron, Link, Wang, and Estes, "Clinical Profile," 118.
6. Talman and Kelkar, "Neural Control of the Heart: Central and Peripheral," *Neurologic Clinics: Neurocardiology* 11:2 (May 1993), 248.

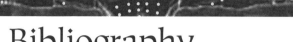

Bibliography

Books

Adams, R., M. Victor, and A. Ropper. 1997. *Principles of neurology*, 6th ed. New York: McGraw-Hill.

Barker, R., J. Burton, and P. Zieve. 1999. *Principles of ambulatory medicine*, 5th ed. Philadelphia: Williams and Wilkins.

Berne, R., and M. Levy. 1999. *Cardiovascular physiology*, St. Louis: Mosby.

Braunwald, E., Z. Douglas, and P. Libb. 1998. *Heart disease: a textbook of cardiovascular medicine*, 5th ed. Philadelphia: Saunders.

Cohen, H. 1999. *Neuroscience for rehabilitation*, 2nd ed. Philadelphia: Lippincott.

DiGiovanna, E., D.O., and S. Schiowitz, D.O. 1991. *An osteopathic approach to diagnosis and treatment*. Philadelphia: Lippincott.

Fauci, A., M.D., E. Braunwald, M.D., K. Isselbacher, M.D., J. Wilson, M.D., J. Martin, M.D., P. Kasper, M.D., S. Hauser, M.D., and D. Longo, M.D. 1998. *Harrison's principles of internal medicine*, 14th ed. New York: McGraw-Hill.

Ganong, W. 1995. *Review of medical physiology*, 17th ed. Norwalk, Conn.: Appleton and Lange.

Hsieh, D. 1995. *Dim mak: the poison hand touch of death*, 9th ed. Taiwan: Meadea Enterprise.

———. 1997. *Advanced dim mak*, 7th ed. Taiwan: Meadea Enterprise.

Kubertur, Henri E., M.D., and G. Franck, M.D. 1999. *Neurocardiology*. Mount Kisco, N.Y.: Futura Publishing Company.

Kuchera, M., D.O., and W. Kuchera, D.O. 1994. *Osteopathic considerations in systemic dysfunction*, 2nd ed. Columbus, Ohio: Greyden Press.

McCarthy, P. 1995. *The bible of karate, bubishi*. Rutland, Vt., Tokyo: Charles E. Tuttle Company, Inc.

Montaigue, E., 1993. *Dim-mak: death point striking.* Boulder, Colo.: Paladin Press.
Netter, F., M.D. 1994. *Atlas of human anatomy.* Summit, N.J.: Ciba-Geigy.
Robbins, S., M.D., V. Kumar, M.D., and R. Cotran, M.D. 1994. *Pathologic basis of disease,* 5th ed. Philadelphia: Saunders.
Rohen, J., and C. Yokochi. 1993. *Color atlas of anatomy,* 3rd ed. New York: Igaku-Shion.
Rowland, L. 1995. *Merrit's textbook of neurology,* 9th ed. Philadelphia: Williams and Wilkins.
Tegner, B. 1968. *Self-Defense nerve centers and pressure points: for karate, jujitsu and atemi waza.* Ventura, Calif: Thor.
Topol, E., and R. Califf. 1998. *Textbook of cardiovascular medicine.* Philadelphia: Lippincott.
Waldman, S., and A. Willie. 1996. *Interventional pain management.* Philadelphia: Saunders.
Wall, P.D., and R. Mcrask. 1989. *Textbook of pain,* 2nd ed. Edinburgh N.Y.: Churchill Livingstone.

Journals
Bleasdale-Barr, K., and C. Mathias. 1998. Neck and other muscle pains in autonomic failure: their association with orthostatic hypotension. *Journ. of the Royal Soc. of Med.* 91(7): 355–359.
Burns, L., D.O. 1907. Visceral-somatic and somato-visceral spinal reflexes. *Journ. of the Amer. Osteopathic Assoc.* 7(2): 54–55.
Curfman, G., M.D. 1998. Fatal impact-concussion of the heart. *New Eng. Journ. of Med.* 338(25): 1841–1843.
Denton, J., and M. Kalelkar. 2000. Homicidal commotio cordis in two children. *Journ. of Foren. Sci.* 45(3): 734–735.
Diehl, R., D. Linden, A. Diehl, and A. Chalkiadaki. 1999. Cerebrovascular mechanisms in neurocardiogenic syncope with and without postural tachycardia syndrome. *Journ. of the Auto. Nerv. Syst.,* 76 (2), 159–166.
Ferrante, L., M. Artico, B. Narducci, and B. Fraioli. (1995) Glossopharyngeal neuralgia with cardiac syncope. *Neurosurg.* 36(1): 58–63.
Galer, B., M.D. 1998. Painful polyneuropathy. *Neurol. Clinics* 16(4): 794.
Gottesman M., B. Ibrahim, A. Elfenbein, A. Mechanic, and S. Hertz. 1996. Cardiac arrest caused by trigeminal neuralgia. *Headache* 36(6): 392–394.
Haker, E., H. Egekvist, and P. Bjerring. 2000. Effect of sensory stimulation (acupuncture) on sympathetic and parasympathetic activities in healthy subjects. *Journ. of the Auto. Nerv. Syst.* 79(1): 52–59.
Kuchta J., A. Koulousakis, A. Decker, and N. Klug. 1995. Pressor and depressor responses in thermocoagulation of the trigeminal ganglion. *Brit. Journ. of Neurosurg.* 12(5): 409–413.
Link, M., M.D., S. Ginsburg, M.D., P. Wang, M.D., J. Kirchhoffer, M.D., C. Berul, M.D., M. Estes, M.D., and Y. Paris, M.D. 1998. Commotio cordis: cardiovascular manifestations of a rare survivor. *Chest* 114(1): 326–328.

BIBLIOGRAPHY

Link, M., M.D., P. Wang, M.D., N. Pandian, M.D., S. Bharati, M.D., J. Udelson, M.D., M. Lee, M.D., M.Vecchiotti, B.S., G. Mirra, M.D., B. Maron, M.D., and M. Estes III, M.D. 1998. An experimental model of sudden death due to low energy chest wall impact (commotio cordis). *New Eng. Journ. of Med.* 338(25): 1805–1811.

Maron, B., M.D., M. Link, M.D., P. Wang, M.D., and M. Estes, M.D. 1999. Clinical profile of commotio cordis: an under appreciated cause of sudden death in the young during sports and other activities. *Journ. of Cardio. Electrophys.* 10(1): 114–120.

Maron, B., M.D., L. Poliac, M.D., J. Kaplan, M.D., and F. Mueller, M.D. 1995. Blunt impact to the chest leading to sudden death from cardiac arrest during sports activities. *New Eng. Journ. of Med.* 333(6) 337–340.

Maron, B., M.D., J. Strasburger, M.D., J. Kugler, M.D., B. Bell, M.D., F. Bradkey, M.D., and L. Poliac, M.D. 1997. Survival following blunt chest impact-induced cardiac arrest during sports activities in young athletes. *Amer. Journ. of Cardiol.* 79(6): 840–841.

Morillo, C., K. Ellenbogen, and P. Fernando. 1997. Pathophysiologic basis for vasodepressor syncope. *Cardiology Clinics: Syncope* 15(2): 233–234.

Natelson, B., M.D., and Q. Chang, B.S. 1993. Sudden death: a neurocardiologic phenomenon. *Neurocardiology* 11(2): 293–294.

Owens, P., and E. O'Brian. Hypotension in patients with coronary artery disease: can profound hypotension cause myocardial ischemic events? *Heart* 82(4): 477.

Samuels, M. M.D. 1993. Neurally induced cardiac damage: definition of the problem. *Neurology Clinics: Neurocardiology* 11(2): 275–287.

Sato A. 1997. Neural mechanisms of autonomic responses elicited by somatic sensory stimulation. *Neurosci. Behav. Phys.* United States 27(5): 610–621.

Sato A., Y. Sato, H. Suzuki, and A. Kimura. 1996. A and C reflexes elicited in cardiac sympathetic nerves by single shock to a somatic afferent nerve include spinal and supraspinal components in anesthetized rats. *Neurosci. Res. Journ.* 25(1): 91–96.

Talman, W., M.D., and P. Kelkar, M.D. 1993. Neural control of the heart: central and peripheral. *Neurol. Clinics* 11(2): 239–256.

Uryvaev I.V., I.B. Iudel'son, and V. Sergeev 1991. Changes in hemostasis and vagal tonus in healthy individuals and patients with facial neuropathy by micro-dose heparin stimulation of nasal receptors. *Vestin Ross Akad. Med. Nauk.* 8: 22-23.

Vincent M., M.D., and H. McPeak. 2000. Commotio cordis: a deadly consequence of chest trauma. *Phys. and Sports Med.* 28(11): 1–5.

Wilkerson, L., D.O. 1997. Martial arts injuries. *Journal of the American Osteopathic Association* 97(4): 221.

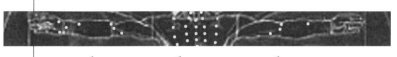

About the Author

Michael Kelly, D.O., attended Rutgers University, where he received a degree in biology, graduated magna cum laude, and was inducted into the Phi Beta Kappa Honor Society. Dr. Kelly received his medical degree from the New York College of Osteopathic Medicine, where he graduated in the top 20 percent of his class. He is currently specializing in internal medicine.

Dr. Kelly worked his way through college while employed as a state police officer. During this time period, he had multiple opportunities to test his martial arts skills and knowledge of dim-mak.

Dr. Kelly began his journey into the martial arts at age 6, when he studied koei-kan karate for a short time. In high school he was involved in competitive wrestling and achieved more than 100 career victories. Now a second-degree black belt in Okinawan shorin-ryu karate, Dr. Kelly has trained in the art for more than 15 years and has had multiple victories in both forms and sparring competitions. In addition, he has studied aikido, tang soo do, and shiatsu. He has been investigating the effects of dim-mak on the body as well as the pressure point attacks hidden within the traditional forms for more than 10 years and has published multiple articles on the medical aspects of dim-mak. This is his first book on the subject.